Classified

Classified

The Secret History of the Personal Column

H. G. Cocks

BOOKS

Published by Random House Books 2009
2 4 6 8 10 9 7 5 3 1

This book includes historical classified advertisements. The information contained in the advertisements is not for current use and should not be relied on under any circumstances. The publisher and author disclaim, as far as the law allows, any liability arising directly or indirectly from the use or misuse of the information contained in this book.

First published in Great Britain in 2009 by
Random House Books
Random House, 20 Vauxhall Bridge Road,
London SW1V 2SA

www.rbooks.co.uk

Addresses for companies within The Random House Group Limited can be found at:
www.randomhouse.co.uk/offices.htm

The Random House Group Limited Reg. No. 954009

A CIP catalogue record for this book is available from the British Library

ISBN 9781847945006

The Ranc
Council (FSC), ...)ur
titles that are ... e
FSC

Typeset

Contents

Introduction

These days, friendship, sex or even love is seemingly only a click away. With the internet it's never been easier or more convenient to meet those who share your interests, however bizarre or mundane, and even to find the man or woman of your dreams. If you do search for the eternal him or her online, you certainly won't be alone. There are more single people in Britain than ever before, and in 2007 the major internet dating sites collectively claimed more than 45 million members in nearly 250 countries, with more than 26 million of those in Britain alone. And that's not even including the 14 million users of Facebook or the 12 million people using teenage networking site Bebo.[1] So instead of working, why not check your Facebook, MySpace or Friendster profile instead, or look at Match.com and Dating Direct to see if you have any fans, potential dates or admirers? We, at least in the industrialised West, and increasingly elsewhere, are all advertisers now.

At least, that's what I thought as I was musing over some long-neglected research, distracting myself with a quick browse through a series of profiles, photos and neat little self-descriptions. It struck me that the personal ad has come a long way. Once regarded as a slightly suspect way of finding the ideal partner – even as an admission of personal failure

– it now seems to be an everyday fact of life. But if we've learned to stop worrying and love the personal ad, when did we overcome our fear and disdain for this eminently practical approach to love and life? And have we really overcome it?

That got me thinking about the personal ad's rise to respectability, and I realised that the file in front of me provided some of the answers. It contained documents dealing with the downfall of one Alfred Barrett, a man who in 1915 was the first to publish a magazine entirely devoted to lonely hearts advertising. His paper, the *Link*, was suppressed in 1921 for 'corrupting public morals'. My initial assumption was that in 1915 meeting the opposite sex via small ads must have appealed to a minuscule number of people. Surely back then most courtship had taken place under the supervision of families, either through the upper class 'season', the rough and ready public encounters of working-class youth, or through the elaborate domestic rituals of middle-class respectability. However, a bit of detective work led me to a whole array of other papers, advertisers, stories and scandals that spanned a huge variety of media and had a past which stretched as far back as the seventeenth century.

At one time, all ads were in the form of short, pithy paragraphs of text, the first of which – a statement of ecclesiastical rules governing the Easter festival – was printed in 1477 by William Caxton.[2] However, ads like these only began to be used to find husbands and wives in the 1690s, around fifty years after the invention of the modern newspaper – the first reference is in the agony column of a periodical called the *Athenian Mercury* in 1692.[3] By the early eighteenth century, matrimonial advertising was booming, along with the expansion of print and the proliferation of newspapers, pamphlets and periodicals.

At first glance, the early advertisements do not seem so different from those that became common in the twentieth century. Men looked for wives, women for husbands, and some even looked for unspecified 'arrangements'. Such was the popularity of these columns that one young lady in 1777 could even complain that 'the mode of advertising is become too general' – although that did not prevent her from placing her own ad, seeking 'a man of fashion, honour, and sentiment, blended with good nature, and a noble spirit, such a one she would chuse for her guardian and protector'.[4] As they have done ever since, these advertisements catered for those slightly at odds with traditional forms of courtship and morality, sometimes women just beyond the customary age of marriage or those distanced from the usual connections of family through the death of parents or by virtue of their own financial independence. In 1827, one such advertiser with independent wealth told her family, who were objecting vigorously to her use of matrimonial papers, that

---

A GENTLEMAN Desirous of Marriage. Gentleman, 25 years of age, and of a healthful constitution, is desirous of altering his condition, by marrying a young lady (or Widow who has no child) and can make a Jointure proportionable to a fortune of 8000 or 10000 l. Advertisements of this kind are often inserted by Gentlemen for their Diversion; I do therefore declare myself in earnest, and the real foundation of applying in this public Way is a Want of Acquaintance in *London* sufficient to introduce me in a private one.

Matrimonial Advertisements, 1750

---

in spite of her brother's strong objections to her suitor, 'she was fully satisfied in her own mind', and 'as she was her own mistress, she should use her own discretion'.[5] Yet although there were thousands of devotees, the anonymity involved – not to mention the necessity of giving chapter and verse on income and prospects in each ad – lent a mercenary air to the whole enterprise and ensured that it was not quite the done thing in polite society.

At the end of the nineteenth century, however, the matrimonial ad gained a new prominence and respectability. With much of Britain's population living in cities by the 1890s, social commentators were becoming concerned that traditional courtship was increasingly outdated. Modern workers, they feared, were spending all their time at the office or in distant suburban lodgings and were finding it hard to meet suitable partners, with the result that some were resorting to the social life of the street and all its illicit temptations. Some respectable journalists, philanthropists and thinkers therefore began to argue that the small ad might be a solution to the difficulties of marriage and the anonymity of modern life. Some even experimented by setting up their own social networks for single people – the first of which was founded in 1898. By the First World War things had progressed a step further. A few enterprising journalists like Alfred Barrett realised that small ads need not serve only those who wanted to marry but also those who were simply looking for companionship. Now you no longer had to say that you were seeking matrimony, just that you wanted a 'pal' or 'companion'. Advertising for 'chums' of both sexes suddenly became fashionable and modern.

Inevitably, lonely hearts ads attracted criticism from those worried that they were a threat to conventional morality. There was some substance to this fear: the personal column did not just cater for people in search of 'ordinary' relationships, it also sheltered those on the edges of law and morality, such as gay men and women, lurking lotharios and adventurous single girls. There was a whole world of correspondence clubs, companionship columns, lonely hearts clubs, dodgy book dealers, matrimonial bureaux, and, by the 1960s, wife swapping societies, who met through the personals. All this was hidden in plain sight between thin lines of type at the back of the newspaper or magazine.

The stories of advertisers, lonely hearts, pornographers, single women and swingers show us how people grappled with the problems and opportunities presented by their often unconventional lives. For them, the personal column was a vital resource, a way of not only making friends and meeting lovers, but also forging a community when homosexuality was still illegal, when being single past the age of twenty-one was seen as embarrassingly shameful, and when the difficulty of obtaining a divorce could make marriage seem like a terrible constraint. From the women advertising for marriage in the 1820s, the single flappers of the 1920s, or the 'artistic' young men of the Edwardian period, right up to the swingers of the 1960s and the children in modern-day chatrooms, the lonely heart and the advertiser have been objects of fascination and concern as emblematic figures of contemporary morality. Collectively, their stories not only tell an oblique history of British morals in the twentieth century, but also plot the long road to respectability taken by the lonely heart.

From small beginnings in magazines like the *Link*, the personal ad (and its modern cousin the internet profile) has become one of the defining features of modern social life and contemporary romance. Its history tells us how ordinary people tried to think their way through homosexuality, pornography, modern marriage, the pleasures and pitfalls of sexual liberation, as well as the gifts and trials of single life. For thousands of advertisers, and for British society as a whole, the small ad was a symbol of everything that was both exciting and dangerous about modern sexuality.

Chapter One

Sporty Girls and Artistic Boys: The Rise and Rise of the Companionship Ad

On 1 September 1920 Sir Basil Thomson, Assistant Commissioner of the Metropolitan Police, received a note warning him of a grave threat to the nation's morals. The letter was from the anti-prostitution campaigner R. A. Bennett, editor of the muck-raking newspaper *Truth*, and enclosed a small pamphlet, available from newsagents in plain cover for the price of 8d. Published monthly, the pamphlet was divided into three advertising sections for 'Ladies', 'Soldiers and Sailors', and 'Civilians', all of whom were seeking 'companions', and 'friends' of both sexes. In addition to the advertisements, which were free, the paper offered a service that would provide up to twelve introductions to other suitable subscribers. This supposed new threat to national morality was called the *Link*, and had been founded in 1915 by an enterprising journalist and former editor of the *Family Circle* named Alfred Barrett. Its front page proudly declared it to be 'The only monthly practically devoted to love interests'. A cursory glance at this publication, Bennett said, would enable the Commissioner to judge its highly immoral character.

Barrett, a suburban journalist on the make masquerading as a metropolitan sophisticate, was a key pioneer of lonely hearts advertising. Although his enterprise had distant ancestors in the seventeenth- and eighteenth-century marriage markets, his paper was the first to be wholly given over to what he called a 'social medium' intended not so much for finding potential spouses but for making dates and 'friendships'. The *Link* also sought to make this type of 'companionship' advertising stylish and lighthearted rather than earnest, solemn and intellectual. The question was, though: was it safe to advertise for companions in this relatively anonymous way, or was it, as the *Link*'s critics argued, the first step on the road to perdition?

BACHELOR GIRL (London W), well-educated, loves books, sunshine, laughter, cinemas, detests Mrs Grundy, orthodoxy, and human cabbages, wants 'really truly' men chums, unconventional, alive. London preferably.

Link, June 1919

Alfred Barrett naturally argued that his paper, whose masthead proclaimed it to be 'helpful, clean, and straight', was nothing but honest and safe. But R. A. Bennett and his moralising ilk clearly thought otherwise. He had studiously gone through the *Link*'s ten pages with a green pencil and marked what he thought were the most dangerous advertisements, underlining the key words and phrases for the benefit of the police. The section devoted to women was, he wrote, 'frank enough', as it seemed to promise adventure with all sorts of 'sporty' or 'jolly' girls, such as the one from 'Bohemian Girl, 24', who was 'interested in most things', and wanted a 'man pal'. Ads such as this, Bennett said, looked foolish but were probably harmless, unlike a number of those placed by men that seemed to be of rather dubious morality and legality. There was, for example, one from 'Iolaus . . . 24', who described himself as 'intensely musical' and of a 'peculiar temperament'. He had, he said, been 'looking for many years for [a] tall, manly Hercules'. Another came from an 'Oxonian . . . 26', also seeking a man pal, who was 'brilliant, courteous, humorous, [a] poet, future novelist, in love with beauty despite cosmic insignificance, [and] masculine'. These coded words, Bennett argued, 'speak for themselves as plainly as such an advertisement could'. As he hardly needed to point out, these advertisers were breaking the law, since not only was sex between men illegal at this time, but so too were any attempts to arrange it. Indeed Bennett had felt prompted to send the paper to the police after hearing about a youth who had made, he said, 'various acquaintances of which his mother strongly disapproves'.

In spite of these objections, the *Link* might have continued and even prospered if it hadn't been for an unfortunate coincidence. Shortly after the police received Bennett's highlighted copy of the *Link* in September 1920, a self-styled bohemian named Walter Birks was arrested in Carlisle on a charge of fraud, and was found to be carrying love letters from one William Ernest Smyth, a 22-year-old clerk living in Belfast. When a police officer visited Smyth's rooms, he discovered evidence of a passionate and lengthy correspondence between the two men, and hundreds of letters from other people. It soon emerged that the correspondence between Smyth and Birks, as well as their subsequent love affair, had been initially arranged via the pages of the *Link*. Some of Smyth's letters were from another clerk – an ex-serviceman named Geoffrey Smith, from Enfield near London. All three advertisers were arrested and charged with conspiring to commit 'gross indecency'. As for Barrett, he was charged with aiding and abetting his advertisers, conspiring to enable the commission of such unnatural acts, and also with the offence of 'corrupting public morals by introducing men to women for fornication'.[1]

The case came to court in June 1921 and was, unfortunately for the defendants, tried by Mr Justice Darling, a pompous martinet and self-appointed scourge of lax post-war morality. Right from the start, the most serious evidence was that of the homosexual ads, many of which came from the personal correspondence of Birks and his lovers. Before this shocking evidence was entered, Darling asked that, owing to the indecent nature of the evidence, two women jurors withdraw and that the public gallery be cleared of people who had no business there. Sir Richard Muir, for the prosecution, said that although women jurors were often useful, in this case no woman, 'except perhaps one off the streets', could even be expected to understand the case. Six young men remained, however, perhaps to hear what was going to happen to their former lovers, friends, and their unwitting patron Alfred Barrett. Darling, who seemed to have made up his mind about the outcome, regarded them sternly. 'When these other people stop and listen to disgusting evidence of this nature', he declared, 'I can hardly distinguish them from those that are guilty, whoever they may be.'[2]

REGGIE (London SE), young bachelor, lonely, affectionate, sincere, musical, theatrical, wishes to meet nice looking young male about 20, if possible share rooms, also week ends. Photo appreciated.

Link, June 1919

Some of the letters between Birks, Smith and their friends

and lovers were certainly incriminating. One in particular recalled a blissful holiday which Birks and his 18-year-old lover 'Vernon' had shared in the Isle of Man in 1919. These prized letters, of which only one has survived, and which Birks had treasured ever since the beginning of their correspondence, recalled fondly that 'we not only shared the same room, My Flower, but the same *bed*'. For Vernon the experience was little short of rapturous. 'Oh heaven!!' he wrote, 'it was indeed "the goods" it was *America*.' He remembered being roused by Birks at 5 a.m. so that they could 'sin again'. But, Vernon mused, had it been a sin? No, it was only sinful 'if to *LOVE* is to sin???' They had simply fallen in love, Vernon concluded, and the consequences were 'only the efforts of *nature* in us asserting her rights!!! [and] we must abide the results!'[3] The disdainful Justice Darling described these passionate missives as 'the most filthy he had ever heard read in a long experience'. They showed, he said, 'a depravity which one could hardly have believed possible'.

While Vernon's rapture shows what resulted from successful advertising, William Smyth's letters, written the following year, tell us something of how men let on that they would be interested in more than just friendship in the first place. All personals have their own codes, and those in the *Link* were no different. The first clear indicator of sexual preference was to establish that you wanted to 'meet chum own sex', as 'Bachelor, 39 . . . affectionate disposition, fond of things in general', put it in 1921. Further, if you described yourself as 'affectionate', 'amiable', 'sincere' or even 'beautiful without vanity', you would certainly catch the eye. You could even, like 'Otherwise Normal', say that you were seeking 'young friends who do not chase girls'. Some of the code words employed were practically clichés. As the police had learned, 'artistic', 'musical', and 'unconventional' all acted as glaring indications of homosexual interest. If the penny still hadn't dropped, a list of authors, playwrights and composers who belonged to a sort of queer artistic canon could be cited in the ads to act as clear statements of intent. Writers such as the Edwardian socialist Edward Carpenter, who had written a number of books about what he called 'the intermediate sex', the American poet of manly comradeship Walt Whitman, and above all Oscar Wilde were consistently mentioned in the *Link*'s pages in order to remove any doubt as to one's interests.

Wilde, who had been imprisoned in 1895 for 'gross indecency', was a key reference point for the male advertisers. His novel of decadent youth, *The Picture of Dorian Gray* (1891), in which the hero lives a life of dissipation and immorality without ever showing it, while his portrait in the attic becomes ever more horribly disfigured, was, as the *Daily Express* noted knowingly, 'mentioned in several letters'. Mr Justice Darling could not resist pointing out the historical parallels to the jury, noting that Wilde's trial had partly turned on the question of whether or not *Dorian Gray* was a homosexual novel.

The Northern Irish *Link* advertiser William Smyth was one of many to adopt an 'artistic' Wildean style. By his own account, he spent hours listening to his favourite music – Schubert, Wagner or Percy Grainger – or gazing at the languorous beauties and lush colours of pre-Raphaelite art. He also had an interest in interiors and was, he wrote to Birks, 'very fond of artistic surroundings, beautiful colours in furniture and curtains and softly shaded lamps and all those beautiful things which appeal to the refined tastes of an artistic mind', namely, 'Flowers, perfume, colour and beautiful scenery'. He concluded by saying that there was 'nothing that I could not give to a friend who loved me' and said that he longed to bestow his love 'in the most intimate way that you could desire'.[4]

Others adopted a more masculine style, including Geoffrey Smith, the Enfield clerk with a distinguished military career, who had met men from as far away as South Shields on Tyneside, where he had been given an engraved signet ring by his lover Frank. The exchange of initialled rings, the police learned, was 'a custom among sodomites' designed to be a 'symbol of their marriage'.[5] If that was not enough to persuade a jury of what was going on behind the pages of the *Link*, evidence could be produced of a Major Lombard ('artistic, musical and literary'), who had asked for introductions to twelve men, and had also sent in a photo of himself dressed as a woman.

The connection between the *Link* and homosexuality seemed clear enough. But was it, as the prosecution argued, also an 'advertisement pimp' which encouraged heterosexual 'fornication' and the prostitution of women? The evidence for that was much thinner. Most of the advertisements placed by women were, on the face of it, tame to say

> Bohemienne, young Southern, sympathetic, intuitive, wide reader, believes in 'naturalness,' worships beauty, seeks congenial correspondents, with view to 'real' friendship. Write fully.
>
> *T. P.'s Weekly*, 26 April 1912

the least. To modern eyes, it would seem that few could have had any objections to the 'Gentlewoman (London, S. W), young widow, very good standing . . . [who] would like to meet cultured man, 30–40'. Still less could moral panic be inspired by the 'Catholic lady (Abroad)', who 'would appreciate letters from gentlemen anywhere in England or Rhine Army'.[6] However, the prosecution argued that amidst the sea of notices placed by innocuous widows there were definitely a number of ads that were pernicious, some of which even seemed to have been placed by married women. One ad introduced at the trial was placed by a 'Young Grass Widow', who frankly admitted that she wished 'to meet [a] straightforward man' in what seemed to be an adulterous quest.

Some of the more obvious heterosexual advertisements were placed by men, such as the 'Lothario, London West, 30', who wanted 'cuddlesome girls', and who was 'fond river, dancing, pleasure'. But other ads were apparently connected to much more serious matters than straightforward seduction, and the prosecution used them to insinuate that women had been put in harm's way and the public's morals corrupted by the promiscuous mixing of the sexes. One ad from 1921 placed by a 'Widow, (London W), greatly interested in discipline', and who wanted to 'hear from others, both sexes', was linked to a woman named Alice Vezey with two convictions for brothel keeping dating back to 1912.[7] Barrett claimed at the time that he knew nothing of this, and had assumed that it represented merely a dispassionate interest in an unusual hobby. Someone could just as easily take an interest in the issue of corporal punishment as they might in capital punishment, he told his readers rather unconvincingly.[8] Two years earlier he had been threatened with prosecution by a man who, via the *Link*, had met and had sex with a woman named Toby Robins. She had then falsely claimed to be pregnant, and had tried to blackmail him. And back in 1916, after only a year in business, Barrett had been warned by the police after somebody had contacted them suggesting that the *Link* ought to be suppressed as it appeared to be 'the official organ of the White Slave Traffic', the melodramatic Victorian euphemism for international prostitution.[9] At the trial the *Link* was even accused of being a kind of white slavers' HQ, and acting as a clearing house for pimps and procurers. At the *Link* offices, the *News of the World* claimed, were discovered bundles of letters which clearly showed 'what the immoral section of the public considered the paper existed for'. These included hundreds of letters 'from women offering to sell their bodies to anyone who came along'. A man had come forward, the press claimed, whose 17-year-old daughter had disappeared, the only clue to her whereabouts being a number of letters from *Link* advertisers.[10]

In court, Barrett admitted that he had been careless with some of the ads, but hadn't realised their 'true character' at the time. The fact was, though, that the very nature of Barrett's business itself put him in an awkward position. Matrimonial advertising, the *Link*'s close relation, had never had a very good reputation. Ever since its earliest days, it had been seen as the last resort of the old, sad and ugly, who were, it was assumed, all vulnerable to the depredations of dishonest marriage brokers. To some observers, Barrett was even worse than his predecessors because his major innovation was to make the *Link* strictly non-matrimonial, unlike his Victorian and Edwardian predecessors in the courtship market. They had rarely deviated from the idea that marriage was the natural aim of their clients, a situation which was reflected in advertisements which made it clear that getting a husband or wife was the desired object. Barrett, however, encouraged the idea that a succession of 'companionships' might be more appealing to his customers and more in tune with contemporary tastes than an immediate statement of marital intent. Accordingly, the *Link* masthead proudly announced it to be 'Social – Not Matrimonial'. It was emphatically not a vehicle for husband-hunting but was instead 'A Monthly Social Medium for Lonely People'.[11] According to its editor, the purpose of the paper was not necessarily to facilitate marriage, but 'to provide a medium by which lonely people can escape from their loneliness, and those in want of friends can be brought in communication with other friendless beings'.[12] 'Immoral relations' might result, but that was no business of the *Link*. Responding to suspicions that the paper might be the agent of seduction, Barrett argued that only evil minds would find evil in the paper. There may be 'risk and danger attending the use of the "Link",' he warned his readers, 'But whereabouts in human relations are they absent?'[13] In his typically avuncular style, Barrett reassured his readers that he vetted all letters personally, and that unsuitable ads would be removed. Danger would result only if readers lent ready and willing aid.[14]

That, then, was the essence of his defence: the *Link* was a wholly respectable enterprise founded as a solution to the epidemic of loneliness which had engulfed modern society.

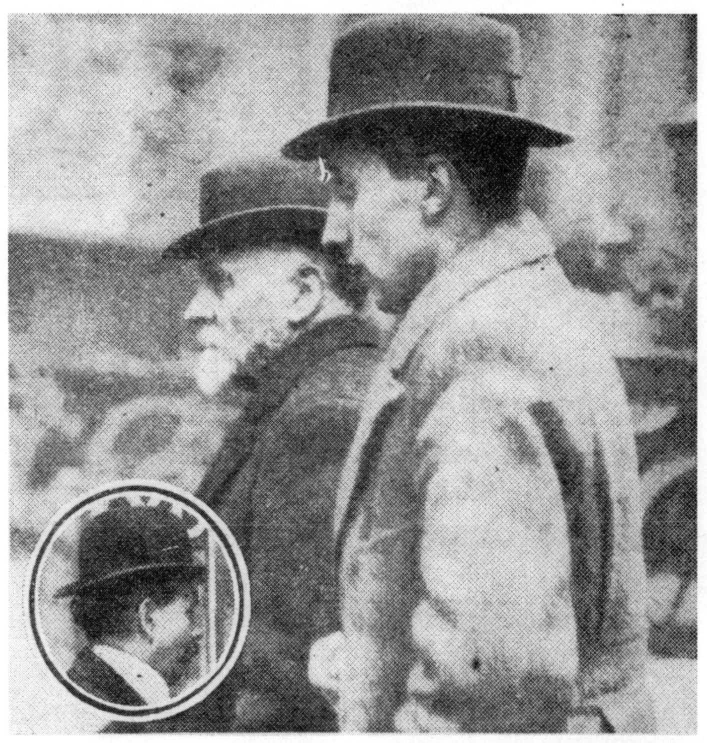

Alfred Barrett (inset), Geoffrey Smith (right) and an unidentified Link *advertiser on their way to be tried for conspiracy to corrupt public morals.*

In his own account, Barrett had founded the *Link* because he had heard of a friend who was returning to Britain after twenty years spent on an Australian ranch. This man's difficulty in meeting members of the opposite sex prompted Barrett to help him out, and led to the thought that 'there must be . . . thousands of such in London alone, to say nothing of the feminine portion of humanity'. The *Link* was therefore not an opportunistic response to the lax wartime moral climate, but was instead fulfilling a long-felt want throughout society.[15] As his barristers pointed out, apart from the disciplinarian Alice Vezey and the innuendoes of the press, the police had failed to provide any evidence of the *Link*'s alleged connection to white slavery. His barristers continually pressed the point that Barrett's paper was not a medium for prostitution but could be proved to be 'a serviceable and useful medium for effecting genuine and sincere friendships', used by respectable 'servant girls, majors, colonels, lawyers, barristers and clergymen'.[16]

Barrett himself was presented by his defence team as the very essence of a respectable editor and novelist. This was, ostensibly at least, what he was. He seemed an unlikely white-slaver. By the time of the trial he was fifty-one years old and had had a long career as a comic novelist and editor of magazines as respectable as the *Christian World*, *Family Circle*, the comic journal *Scraps*, and the women's paper *Mary Bull*, which he had left to set up the *Link*. The only known photograph of him shows a bowler-hatted and wing-collared Edwardian gent, going to his doom with, one hopes, his characteristic air of insouciance. Yet for all his extensive writings, Barrett remains a man of mystery. For someone so prolific – he wrote more than fifty books – he has left little record of his life, and rarely said anything about himself. On the surface, he lived a blameless suburban life in Balham, from where he took the train every day to his office in Fleet Street. In several of his stories, he wrote about the joys of home, marriage and fatherhood, its little dramas, trials and wonders. In dedicating a book to his wife, 'whose comfortable and encouraging appreciation has made me alive to the unsuspected advantages of having a critic on the hearth', he conjured up the very image of companionable domesticity.[17] Yet his fiction is full of doppelgangers, double lives and parallel universes. Did he, like the characters in his stories, also lead a sort of double life? His work seemed to require it, forcing him to leave behind the persona of suburban husband as he disembarked at Waterloo, to exchange it for the garb of the louche gentleman journalist.

Perhaps there was another reason, too, why Barrett seemed obsessed with doubleness and imposture. Was there a hint that it was his own sexual ambiguity which made him less than particular about the ads of 'musical' young men? On the surface it seems unlikely, but when the police raided his house in the spring of 1921, they discovered an interesting cache. Under Barrett's bed lay not only about 100 indecent photographs, but also a collection of French pornography relating to 'abominable practices', a ponderous Victorian euphemism for homosexual acts.[18] Mr Justice Darling had no doubt that Barrett had more than a professional interest in his paper, and conjured up a lurid vision of the depraved corrupter of public morals poring over his private collection, lost in homosexual reverie.

Making the Lonely Hearts Industry

Whatever the truth about Barrett, he was certainly not the only one trying to make money out of lonely vicars, lovesick housemaids and fans of Walt Whitman. In 1915, when the *Link* was launched, it was actually operating in a fairly crowded market, competing against various solidly respectable papers, journals and clubs, all of which were trying to capture the contemporary fad for 'palling up'. All were anxious to stress their respectability and to combat suspicions that personal ads were merely for the mercenary or the gullible. In fact, the lonely hearts business had its origins in a kind of experiment in social networking which not only proclaimed the most impeccable moral credentials but also built in a number of safeguards against immorality. We think of networks like MySpace or Facebook as inherently modern inventions, dependent on the immediacy of contemporary technology, but they were actually invented in 1898, and relied on the more mundane ministrations of the Post Office. The campaigning editor W. T. Stead, who was also virtually the inventor of modern journalism with all its sensationalism and banner headlines, was the first to set up such a network in order to try and facilitate marriage between the thousands of young men and women adrift in the anonymous modern city. While Barrett saw the untapped potential in the companionship ad, and made it more popular and contemporary, Stead started his social network, the Wedding Ring Circle, as a respectable method of encouraging middle-class marriage.

Stead's Circle relied on a growing feeling that in the anonymous modern city, traditional middle-class courtship, which relied on introductions to the family home, was increasingly inadequate. Bourgeois writers complained that while other classes had their own tried and tested methods of organising relations between the sexes, such as the aristocratic 'season' or the free and easy 'monkey parade' promenading of working-class youth, there was nothing specifically designed for them. The young men and women of the middle class, increasingly immured in offices during the day, and spending their evenings in poky rooms in distant suburbs, required their own, new means of interaction.

> B. 78. Middlesex – Age 25; fair, slight, fond of music, and a lively temperament; would like to make the acquaintance of an educated, refined man not under 30; not necessarily for marriage; wishes to correspond with a gentleman who is cultured and of a sympathetic disposition, either a business or professional man, but must be at least 30, and not more than 50; not a clergyman; a man of broad views and fond of music.
>
> *Round-About*, 2 July 1898

For 12s and 6d, or 17s if living abroad, you could join the Wedding Ring Circle (soon renamed the Correspondence Club) to look for a husband, wife or friend. Before long, the club had outgrown its mainly matrimonial purpose and the section for those seeking 'intellectual friends' of the opposite sex had taken over the enterprise. In this first effort at dating the English way, each member filled in a form in which they described briefly their personality and their requirements. They then received the WRC's monthly magazine, *Round-About*, and had access to the photograph album containing members' pictures, and the autograph album containing their thoughts on 'the subject that interests them most'. The albums were held centrally at the *Round-About* office in London, where the 'Controller' of the club vetted all letters and advertisements. Members could also form 'manuscript journals', in which small groups exchanged thoughts on whatever they decided to discuss, from 'social questions', to the Welsh. The idea was that friendship would result without the strain and anxiety of courtship. Members retained their anonymity throughout all correspondence, and the Controller only revealed their identity with the consent of both parties when they were perfectly satisfied with their companion's *bona fides*.

At roughly the same time, the companionship ad became popular with much more radical thinkers. Socialist and anarchist advocates of 'free love' (which usually meant common-law marriage or any kind of union that did not have the sanction of the law) began to see the lonely hearts ad as a way not only of remaking society but also of safeguarding the future of the British race. This kind of thinking owed a lot to eugenics, the pseudo-science of racial improvement. At that time, it was common on the left to advocate eugenic measures, not in the Nazi sense of extensive state murder, but as part of a programme of progressive social reforms. In the 1890s, intellectuals and commentators worried that the very poorest, who in their view were most likely to succumb to disease and depravity, were reproducing faster than the healthy and moral. This 'degeneration' of the population could be combated by a series of measures designed to improve public, and by extension racial, health. While some of the suggestions, such as compulsory sterilisation, were undoubtedly coercive, others were impeccably progressive, and included proposals for social welfare, unemployment insurance and maternal healthcare.

The idea of 'racial health' formed part of the background of many political ideas at the end of the nineteenth century, and the companionship ad was one unlikely, yet popular, manifestation of this trend. Its intellectual origins even owed something to Charles Darwin's writings on animal courtship and evolution. Many radical socialists had taken notice of Darwin's contention that racial health was promoted by what he called 'mate competition', that is, the ability of female animals to choose their partners. The chief obstacle to this form of selection in human societies was class. Free-love theorists argued that if men and women could get round the barriers of class which kept healthy people apart, then this kind of mate competition would act as an evolutionary mechanism. As a consequence, healthy and racially 'fit' people would be able to meet, marry and have children, thereby promoting racial fitness in a natural manner. In this way, they would not only destroy the conventions which held back social reform, but also produce healthier babies and make Britain a stronger and better place.[19]

Eugenics, socialism, free love and the lonely hearts ad consequently became somewhat unlikely bed-fellows. In 1897 a short-lived magazine of socialist free love, the *Adult* (1896–99) carried lonely hearts advertising which encouraged men and women to break the bonds of custom and meet better partners from outside their class. This would enable people to base their free union not on the stale requirements of respectability, but on compatibility alone. Radical social experimentation was the end, lonely hearts ads were the means. At least we have to assume that that was the real object of one typical *Adult* advertiser, a 'Young gentleman (29), dark, tall, with literary tastes', who desired 'correspondence with young blonde. Photo in confidence'.[20]

Both the Wedding Ring Circle and the *Adult* required substantial commitment – the former to intellectual debate and correspondence, and the latter to a difficult brand of radical politics. There was obviously a gap in the market for a less onerous kind of club. It was filled by a literary journal called *T. P.'s Weekly*, founded in 1902 and named after its editor and proprietor, the veteran pressman and Irish Nationalist politician Thomas Power O'Connor. *T. P.'s Weekly* contained two columns, 'NQA' (Notes, Queries and Answers) and 'Friends in Council Queries', both of which grew gradually into a forum for lonely hearts ads.

A Lady, who is naturally rather quiet, but at the same time likes a little amusement, is anxious to make the acquaintance of another who would go out with her occasionally to café or theatre in London.

T. P.'s Weekly, 2 January 1914

By 1911 *T. P.'s*, then being edited by the socialist bohemian Holbrook Jackson, had developed its 'Friends in Council' section into the most popular companionship column in Britain. In the five years to 1915, over 8,000 ads appeared and the paper claimed to be dealing with 500–600 letters a week, or about 31,000 a year.[21] Typical advertisers in those early years included modern young women ('Bright Cheero Girls'), countless 'refined bachelors', thousands of servicemen and a selection of 'lonely colonials', all looking for correspondents, mainly of the opposite sex. They shared column space with a huge variety of advertisers, from Parisian ladies interested in literature and art to the 'Rolling Stone, Gentleman', who sought 'chummy correspondents', especially ladies with an artistic temperament.[22]

'Friends in Council' rapidly overflowed with similar advertisements priced at 1d per word. However, the paper was never as bold as Barrett's *Link* in proclaiming a new morality and it initially tried to stop people using the columns to make dates and companionships. Perhaps paradoxically, in the light of what happened to the *Link*, the editors at first tried to guarantee the morality of the column by restricting ads to those seeking their own sex.[23] However, this restriction only ensured that certain ads flourished that would only a few years later seem suspicious and even blatant. For instance, 'Friends in Council' opened 1914 with the announcement that a student of Whitman and Carpenter from Sheffield, who styled himself 'Calamus' after Whitman's homoerotic verse, was 'desirous of getting in touch with anyone living in district similarly interested'.[24] Many other similar ads appeared from sincere young men.

Busy Bachelor Girl (London), sincere and refined, usual social accomplishments, interested in others, and perhaps a little interesting herself, would appreciate a correspondence from gentlemen over thirty or similar dispositions, with view to friendship. Replies strictly confidential.

T. P.'s Weekly, 2 January 1914

Although opposite-sex ads were initially regulated, homosexual contacts like this continued with impunity, and by

1914 the moral regulations governing other advertisements in *T. P.'s Weekly* had been similarly liberalised, although with some suitable precautions in place. In particular, the ban on contacting the opposite sex had been dropped, and such companionships could now be requested as long as the advertiser provided two references to character, one of which had to be from a clergyman. An additional condition attempted to regulate the morality of the column by banning the words 'broad-minded' and 'unconventional' which meant 'so much or so little to various readers', from all advertisements. Requests for photographs were also disallowed, because it smacked too much of the introduction agency, and 'if intellectual friendship is desired what matters the appearance or station of the correspondent [?]'.[25] In addition to these services, *T. P.'s Weekly* ran the Circle Correspondence Club, through which subscribers (at the rate of 1s for three months) could retain their anonymity in the early stages of a correspondence. In spite of all the fears raised by the *Link* trial, in 1914 the world of 'companionship' seemed safe and respectable.

The End of the *Link*

The fact that the new trend for dating had influential and respectable – albeit less daring – friends, as well as the backing of large numbers of ordinary men and women, did not, however, save Alfred Barrett and his co-defendants. In spite of all the evidence testifying to the popularity of the lonely hearts ad, the laws punishing male homosexuality were emphatically against them. On 8 June 1921, Barrett was found guilty of corrupting public morals, and of aiding and abetting his advertisers in a conspiracy to procure acts of gross indecency. The other men were found guilty of conspiring to commit the acts of gross indecency. There could be no greater attack on the morals of the country, Mr Justice Darling told Barrett, than to 'establish a paper as you did for the purpose of allowing men and women to commit immorality'.[26] Regretting bitterly that he could not dispatch the defendants to penal servitude, Darling settled for the scarcely less onerous maximum sentence: two years' imprisonment with hard labour. Soon afterwards, several papers began to reconsider the wisdom of carrying companionship ads. The risqué bachelor weekly *London Life*, which had been running a 'Do You Want a Pal?' column since 1918, had clearly watched the trial with trepidation, and quietly pulled the plug on its lonely hearts columns. Barrett, who had done so much to make the lonely hearts ad a feature of modern life, was lost to history, probably returning after his prison sentence to suburban obscurity and years of anonymous and decreasingly profitable scribbling for anyone who would take it. His hour in the limelight was over. But had the companionship ad met a similarly untimely end?

Chapter Two

Lonely Soldiers

The downfall of Barrett and the *Link* seemed like the end for the companionship ad, but this was far from the case. He had, in fact, tapped into a vibrant contemporary trend: a yearning for a more casual and fashionable way of courtship, something that required neither an elaborate social ritual nor a formal introduction to the middle-class home. This trend was no better illustrated than by the story of Barrett's wartime competitors who entered the lonely hearts market under the guise of patriotic service. For just as Barrett was starting the *Link*, he was joined in the companionship business by a series of papers seeking to comfort and console the thousands of soldiers, sailors and airmen fighting across Europe and the Empire, and who together fuelled a boom in what was called 'lonely soldier' correspondence. The arrival of war in 1914, and the absence of large numbers of men from home, ensured that packages, gifts and letters were soon being sent to the forces in enormous numbers. By the end of 1914, these lonely soldiers were also advertising in the press for correspondents, pals, and perhaps more. Famous actresses and forces' favourites got involved, even offering to marry the right man. Before long, though, the War Office noticed that hundreds of thousands of letters were being exchanged between complete strangers and military personnel, and began to worry about the threat to national security that such missives might encourage.

To begin with, sending 'breezy correspondence' to a lonely soldier was presented as a patriotic duty, one way of linking the home front with the war and of allowing men and women at home to claim a role in the conflict, even if it was only one of comfort and consolation. The *Daily Chronicle* was one of the first to try it, supplying two battalions serving in France, some 1,800 men, with Christmas gift boxes of tobacco, cigarettes, chocolate and peppermints, all provided by their readers at a cost of 5 shillings per man. Supplying the troops with the comforts of home was not a million miles away from offering them consolation by letter, and soon soldiers were advertising for correspondence and pals, just like their civilian counterparts in *T. P.'s Weekly* and the *Link*.

Lonely soldiers not only represented an almost unending source of pals and potential husbands, but were also an ideal propaganda opportunity. Their letters could be used to show that, even while doing their patriotic duty, men at the front were always thinking of the homes they were defending. It was not long before being a lonely soldier could even make you a celebrity. In the spring of 1915, the *Daily Express* claimed to have found, in Private A. C. White of the 1st Rifle Brigade, 'the loneliest man at the front'. In the run-up to the war, the *Express* had briefly run its very own *Link*-style 'Lonely Men's League' as a solution to modern isolation, and White was recommended for its aid by his friend, Private Dowdall. Rifleman White's story was a tragic one, Dowdall said. His comrade was an orphan who had lied about his age to enlist, but since he had no family he had 'not received a letter or a parcel since he has been out here; nor is he likely to in the future, for he has no friends'. There was no one who cared sufficiently to send the slightest word of encouragement to him. '"I don't mind as a rule",' White told his companion, 'his eyes grown curiously bright in the candle light and a break in his voice that belied his words, "but when I see the other chaps with their letters an' parcels full o' things to eat, I feel . . ." He did not tell me what he felt, but I knew.' White was in hospital with 'nerves and general weakness', and although, Dowdall said, 'they are doing their best to cure him with pills', it was not pills he needed, but 'a little human sympathy'.[1]

Within two days White had received 470 letters and 200 parcels. Barely a week later, the Rifleman had received over 800 presents, newspapers and boxes, 'almost enough to set him up for life as a grocer, confectioner, and newsagent!' His haul included fifteen tuck boxes, thirty glasses of potted meat, fifteen tins of Milkmaid Café au Lait, fifteen packets of nut-milk chocolate, fifteen tins of smoked sardines, fifteen tins of herring in tomato, fifteen tins of Oxford sausages, fifteen pots of campaigning Bovril, seven and a quarter pounds of ginger chips, several pounds of mixed drops, and fifteen tin-openers. From being the loneliest man in the forces, he was now the 'most hustled and "lionised" man in the brigade, with troops of friends in the Old Country'. The episode united Home Front with Western Front, and, according to the *Express*, was a valuable

Someone, somewhere on active service, would welcome correspondents, opposite sex, in an exchange of opinions, other than war topics.

T. P.'s Weekly, 12 February 1916

contribution to the war effort. One of the paper's patriotic soldier correspondents declared that the lonely soldier movement showed that 'though everything is going well with the Allies, the sympathy of the British public is great'.[2]

In the French army, lonely soldier advertising was even more popular and also overlapped with the emerging lonely hearts market. There, the French state helped to organise lonely soldier advertising, and any moral objection there might have been to anonymous correspondence between men and women was felt to be outweighed by the need to maintain morale. Letters to the men at the Front were explicitly promoted as one way for women to participate in the national struggle by offering their love and perhaps something more as a contribution to the war effort.[3] The correspondents were known as *marraines de guerre* (godmothers of war) and performed what was originally envisaged as a quasi-maternal role of consolation and comfort to their *filleuls* (adopted sons). However, for all its connotations of duty and patriotism, such advertising soon became the way for soldiers to strike up friendships with women whom they could pursue when on leave.[4] At the Front, where soldiers remained stuck in trenches and dugouts for days and weeks at a time, letters, gifts and adverts offered the hope of escape from the reality of war. Some commentators even felt that these missives might in themselves be pregnant with sexual meaning. The great German sexologist Magnus Hirschfeld, whose *Sexual History of the Great War* pointed out that sex was a weapon in the conflict, and that soldiers on all sides rarely thought about anything else, noted that every combatant nation had organised some kind of lonely soldier advertising. He maintained that this kind of correspondence was inherently sexualised. For the frontline soldier immured in a dugout, 'a tiny gift from home, sent by some beloved hand, would', he reasoned, 'have a very definite erotic value and significance'.[5]

By 1915, British lonely soldier advertising was established in the *Link*, *T. P.'s Weekly* and much of the mainstream press. While many of the ads were ostensibly asking only for pen pals and chums, they could easily be turned to other purposes. Soon, many of the lonely soldier columns were serving the requirements of lonely hearts, both servicemen and civilians, with *T. P.'s Weekly* and the *Link* functioning as the principal outlet for this type of ad. Many advertisers were anxious to make it clear that they did not want merely sisterly concern. The 'Lonely Subaltern, 25, up to his neck in Flanders mud', who advertised in *T. P.'s* in February 1916, and who 'would welcome cheery correspondence from [a] cheery refined girl with a view [to] friendship', was typical. He was clearly becoming bored with general expressions of concern, though, and 'gratefully declined advice for the prevention of bronchitis'.[6] Others, such as 'Lonely Officer' looking for cheerful girl correspondents, stipulated that 'killjoys' were barred from responding and specified 'no cigarettes, mufflers or Balaklava helmets'. Even displaced Belgian soldiers advertised.[7]

Lonely Young Officer, up to his neck in Flanders mud, would like to correspond with young lady (age 18–20), cheery and good looking.

T. P.'s Weekly, 12 February 1916

Fans of these lonely soldiers varied from the usual troops of sporty girls to the more rarefied, sincere and musical young men who later got the *Link* into so much trouble. Some advertisers were particularly keen on certain branches of the service, including one 'Modern Girl', who wanted to correspond with a 'naval officer (submarine preferred)'. A 'Young Man' was looking for 'male chum, 17–23, London, soldier or sailor preferred', while others were themselves ex-servicemen, such as 'Billy . . . late RN', 'looking for correspondence with own sex', or 'Bachelor, just discharged, intelligent, artistic temperament, though rather pagan', who wanted 'friends, own sex'.[8]

Two wartime novels give us an idea of how lonely soldier correspondence might have worked in practice. *April's Lonely Soldier* by S. P. B. Mais tells the story of two wartime pen pals who correspond, meet and finally fall in love, although they do not get married. April, 22, has just been sent down from Cambridge and, in common with so many modern women, has a tedious office job and lives alone in dingy lodgings. So when she sees an ad placed in *The Times* by 'lonely Subaltern, witty, cheerful, intellectual', she sees a chance for diversion. At first, she worries that he is doing it as a joke and is 'likely to be one of a band of young "bloods" whose sole object is to pull the leg of some unfortunate young girl like myself by decoying her into writing stupid nonsense which you can proclaim on the housetops'.[9] April nevertheless decides to treat him as the ideal companion and to write to him as if he 'were just that friend for whom I have been looking in vain all my life, to whom I may unburden my lonely heart'.[10] She arranges to meet him, adopting an alter ego called Betty just to be on the safe side, but she soon drops the pretence and they of course fall in love.

Dorothy Black's *Her Lonely Soldier* (1916) is more morally

ambiguous as Cicely the heroine is already married to an aged industrialist. She carries on what amounts to an extra-marital courtship with one Captain MacIntosh, a lonely officer with no family. When he is wounded and loses his memory she nurses him back to health and prompts the return of his senses by writing down her name and address, which he recalls from their long correspondence. Eventually they are married, Cicely's husband having conveniently died in the meantime. Although Cicely and April express some reservations about writing to strange men, in both novels the lonely soldier ad is presented as helpful and even moral. It is seen as a uniquely female contribution to the care of the soldier, wounded or otherwise.

Getting in Trouble: Actresses, Lonely Soldiers and the War Effort

In time, however, the enormous popularity of lonely soldier advertising began to trouble the military authorities. In the first place, they worried that its sheer volume was threatening to swamp the army postal system. 'By yesterday's mail from England', Captain T. P. Hobbins of the Royal Engineers complained in February 1915, one Driver Pennery of the Field Artillery had received three sacks, one containing about 3,000 letters, and two more full of small parcels and packets along with 98 other parcels. It turned out that Pennery had advertised as a lonely soldier in the *Daily Chronicle*. Transport problems at the front were bad enough, the Captain said, without this additional burden, and if any more men in the battery received this amount of correspondence 'the transport and disposal of the mails would be seriously hindered'.[11] Moreover, as the Secretary of the Post Office put it, the generosity of respondents would only alert a lonely soldier's comrades to this source of largesse. When more soldiers realised 'the gullibility of the British public', the system would, it was assumed, be inundated with sacks and parcels on the way to the trenches.[12]

The military authorities were also concerned that advertising for correspondence might also end up helping the enemy. The War Office conjured up a vision of battalions of Mata Haris combing through the classifieds and enticing British soldiers to reveal military details. To prevent this the government issued a D-notice to the press in May 1916 warning them 'to refrain from publishing letters and advertisements inviting officers and men in the field to communicate with strangers' or including 'appeals to the public from members of the Expeditionary Force for correspondence, gifts or loans'. The problem, it was claimed, was that enemy agents, 'especially women', were 'taking advantage of the practice that has grown up of encouraging correspondence between the troops and strangers and are through this means collecting information regarding the number and position of the Allied forces'.[13]

There was a medical aspect to all this as well: the authorities were concerned that military effectiveness and the health of soldiers might be impaired by the ever-present threat of VD that might accompany the sort of casual encounters for which some advertisers seemed to be searching. One letter in particular, in response to an ad in the *People* newspaper ('Young lady would like to correspond with a lonely Tommy'), was singled out as an example of how soldiers could get into trouble with anonymous women. Almost none of the millions of lonely soldier letters have survived, but this one at least indicates that servicemen were looking for a little more than motherly consolation. 'Dear Miss', wrote Lance Corporal J. Mullaney of the Medical Corps in October 1916 in reply to the young lady, 'I would like to correspond with you, with the hope of meeting you . . . on some future date. Write immediately.' He signed off warmly, if not suggestively: 'Bon nuit mon chere xxxxxx. I would like to have your photo I will send you one of mine in return, Good bye dear xxxx write soon. ps send me your home address.'[14]

Two Solitary Sister Susies, tired of sewing shirts for soldiers, would like to correspond with two lonely Colonial officers, or gentleman rankers. Fond of music, country life and sport. Ages 25 and 29.

T. P.'s Weekly, 12 February 1916

One particular event seems to have finally snapped military patience with the lonely hearts industry. In the summer of 1916, *Pearson's Weekly* teased soldiers and civilians alike with a competition in which the prize was a series of dates with the actress and soldiers' pin-up Phyllis Monkman. The set-up was that she was looking for her ideal man, perhaps even for a husband. 'Who will marry Phyllis Monkman?' the paper asked, promising 'A chance for single men'.[15] The competition went in four stages, the first consisting of filling in a form describing yourself. The actress would then pick fifty to correspond with, from whom six would be chosen for a personal introduction. From these six, Miss Monkman would select the man who most closely approximated her ideal. If he matched up, she would marry him.

The idea was perfectly calculated to appeal to lonely servicemen. Monkman claimed to have come up with the scheme herself when sifting through fan letters which came in their thousands from the Front. One of these contained a beloved and battered picture of her that a fan had found in the debris of a dugout after the battle of Loos. Seeing this pathetic memorial, Monkman wondered if it would be possible to console the troops, encourage the war effort, and even to meet her ideal man simply by sorting through her many admirers. Thousands of competition entries poured in over the next two weeks, many from 'our fine fellows who are fighting out in France and hoping they'll be the lucky ones'.[16] Monkman replied to them in her weekly column, promising that she was thinking of all the lonely soldiers and sailors, and enlisting romance in the service of wartime propaganda. Many of the letters, she noted, were from wounded men who had done their share in the Big Push on the Somme and who were now 'resting in Blighty, getting fit to go back and punish the Huns some more'.[17]

Whatever propaganda value Phyllis Monkman's lonely hearts escapade may have had, it ultimately exasperated the military authorities and the competition was terminated before she could find her ideal or any lonely soldiers could call her marital bluff. In the same summer of 1916, as the army dealt with the disastrous consequences of the massive Somme offensive, four papers in all were warned off publishing lonely soldier ads or running competitions which 'undoubtedly aimed at men getting into trouble with unknown people in this

Who Will Marry Phyllis Monkman?

A Chance for Single Men.

WOULD you marry Phyllis Monkman if you had the chance?

Perhaps she wouldn't want to marry you—perhaps she would.

Anyway, she can't do so unless she knows you. And she can't know you unless she meets you. And she can't meet you unless you get an introduction.

That's where *Pearson's Weekly* comes in. As you will see if you read the article on the next column, Miss Monkman is in search of her Ideal Man—that is, a man who comes most nearly to her ideal.

Your Editor believes that such a man exists amongst his readers, and is willing to prove it. In order to do so, he asks your aid.

There will be four clearly defined stages in the process of selection.

THE FIRST STAGE.

We invite all single men who would like Miss Phyllis Monkman as a wife, to fill up the form below, and send it to us together with any further statement they may care to make in order to urge their suit.

SECOND STAGE.

Miss Monkman will make a selection of fifty, who will be communicated with by letter.

THIRD STAGE.

From these fifty, Miss Monkman will ultimately choose six, and these six will have the privilege of a *personal introduction*.

FOURTH STAGE.

From amongst these six Miss Monkman will then pick out the man she considers she would like to know better, since he approaches most nearly to her ideal. If the fortunate man actually fulfils Miss Monkman's ideal, then she will marry him.

Who is going to be the happy man? Why should it not be You?

Fill up the form below, and you may be chosen as one of those who will at least have the pleasure of a *personal introduction to Miss Monkman*.

If you are one of the fifty, you will receive from her a large photograph of herself *signed by her*.

Sailors, soldiers, and civilians are all eligible. Now, if you are free to marry, be a suitor, and fill up the form below, *which must be used in applying*.

P.W.—July 8.15.

Age.................... *Height*....................

Weight....................

Colour of Hair....................

" " *Eyes*....................

Clean-shaven or Moustache....................

Trade or Profession....................

If fond of Sport....................

Favourite Recreation....................

Name....................

Address....................

....

HOW THE IDEA CAME.

By PHYLLIS MONKMAN.

THE call-boy had just informed me that the curtain was "up," so I struggled into my first dress and prepared to open a bunch of letters, smoke a cigarette, and talk a little before starting my evening's work.

"Lots of letters from the Front?" asked a visitor casually—a journalist, by the way.

"Heaps! They write to me so often and so cheerfully from the trenches and the sea," I had to admit. "Oh! here's something rather interesting."

I unhooked a large picture of myself from above my dressing-table. It was a battered picture in a plain wooden frame that had once been white. The glass had gone, the frame was scratched and dirty and broken, and right across the picture were furrows and splashes, dull-red in colour.

"It came to me the other day," I told my visitor, "straight from the trenches. An officer posted it to me, with a letter, saying he had found it buried under the *débris* of a dug-out near Loos. It had evidently been through a very fierce battle. Look at the bullet-marks and those unmistakable stains! So he thought I might like to keep it as a curious souvenir."

We gazed at it silently, and as I looked at my name written across the picture I couldn't help wondering where, when, and in what light-hearted moment I had signed that photograph, and who the owner had been? I don't suppose I shall ever know. . . . There was something almost uncanny in this feeling of the Finger of War, right in the midst of a theatre dressing-room, with its bright lights, and paint and powder and artificiality.

Then, to cap our serious thoughts, in came a girl I have known for many years, looking—oh, so sad!

"Men are horrid beasts," she began without preamble. "Just horrid! You remember——? Well, I thought he was my ideal man—the best and finest man in the world—the only man I would like for a husband. And now he's disappointed me beyond words. He's not my ideal man at all. It's too awful!"

We sympathised; and, carelessly, I said: "I wonder if any girl really finds her ideal man?"

"Well, does any girl *know* what her ideal is in mankind?" put in the journalist.

"I do!" I replied quickly. "I do, indeed! I've got my ideal fixed in my mind, but whether he exists or not, I don't know. Probably not."

"Of course not!" sighed my disillusioned friend. "And if he does, once you'd found him you'd discover he wasn't your ideal at all—like me!"

Ungrammatical, but unhappy, she stared gloomily at me; and I began to feel the world was indeed a desert full of girls searching wildly for their ideal man, and never finding him. How is it possible to find him when the world is so wide, and each girl meets comparatively few men in her journey through life? An ideal man—how to find him? Suppose for a wild instant he existed. What a problem! Then I looked at my bunch of letters from men I have probably never seen, and I wondered if one of them might prove to be my ideal man—if ever I had a chance to find out.

"Every single girl forms her own idea of a perfect man and a perfect husband," I protested. "And I expect he exists somewhere or other. Wouldn't it be splendid to find him?"

"Why don't you try?" said the journalist.

"How?" was my amazed query.

"By a competition. If I can find a paper to take up the idea, will you go through with it?"

I was interested. "What must I do?" I asked.

"Choose your ideal man from a big bunch of competitors, who will send in particulars about themselves, for a competition. If among thousands of readers your ideal man exists, it is for you to say you have found him. Will you do it?"

I said "Yes." And the very next day I heard that *Pearson's Weekly* would start this competition; and you will find all the particulars in this number. Curious, wasn't it? And exciting, too, for that's the true story of "How It Began."

Photo, Rotary Photographic Co.

PHYLLIS MONKMAN, the charming actress and dancer, who is in search of her Ideal Man.

Actress and soldiers' pin-up Phyllis Monkman advertises for a husband. The publicity stunt proved too much for the military authorities.

country'.[18] The *People, Pearson's Weekly* and *My Pocket Novels* were all served notice to stop publishing lonely soldier ads, while the *Cambria Daily Leader* of Swansea and the *Sheffield Weekly Telegraph* were told to wind up their war correspondence clubs. At the same time, Alfred Barrett's *Link* began to be scrutinised by the police. The authorities also tried to stop soldiers from putting ads in newspapers, corresponding with strangers or asking for gifts. Even in normal correspondence, the directive said, 'the greatest care must be taken to avoid giving information of military value' and as a result 'playing into the hands of the enemy spy system'.[19]

Lonely Australian Officer, Varsity education, age 25, at present in Flanders desires correspondence from some cheerful soul on any old subject.

T. P.'s Weekly, 12 February 1916

Yet even this official hostility did not kill off the lonely soldier ad. It simply moved it away from the mainstream press who now thought twice about trying to marry off actresses. Soldiers and sailors, lonely or otherwise, gay or straight, continued to advertise in the less obvious pages of the *Link*, *T. P.'s Weekly* and other racy journals like the bachelor periodical *London Life*. It seemed that the lonely hearts ad was here to stay.

Although companionship ads now moved across to 'less respectable' publications, by 1918 the mainstream press retained a charitable view of lonely soldiers and their chums, and of the lonely hearts industry that they supported. The *Sunday Pictorial* praised the companionship ad as a remedy for the 'state of loneliness in which so many English men and women live'. The *Daily Chronicle*, which had pioneered the lonely soldier movement and also ran its own 'Good Fellowship Club', similarly wrote approvingly of the *Link*, 'a little periodical with which possibly everyone but myself is already acquainted'.[20] Given the melancholy state of modern courtship, with overly regimented middle-class couples on one side, and anarchic wartime immorality on the other, it was scarcely surprising that the national press began to recommend the *Link* as at least the beginnings of a response.

As Armistice Day came and went, the *Link* and the lonely soldier movement started to epitomise a new, post-war spirit among those who, as Wilfred Owen put it, had 'seen all things red', and who wanted to forget the war as quickly as possible. This was the generation that embraced the casual, breezy and brittle sensibility of the 'roaring twenties', and who found the companionship ad to be the ideal medium for the expression of this new feeling. Consequently, even though there was no longer a need to console lonely servicemen, and although the *Link* was to be buried by scandal and its editor imprisoned, companionship ads continued to appear, often in the most unlikely places. *Link*-style companionship advertisements seeking friends of one's own sex, and often specifying physical appearance, offering holiday companionships with expenses paid and the exchange of photographs appeared even in the *Daily Express* until at least the mid-1920s.[21] Cheap pulp magazines ran their own 'Lovecraft Clubs' in which modern youth palled up or argued about modern morals. Even the body-building paper *Health and Strength* started a 'League of Physical Culture' as a kind of personal column in which its muscular readers could write for friendship. Recognising this new spirit, at least one matrimonial agent developed a 'platonic branch' for men and women unready to commit themselves to matrimony.

By the early 1920s, many commentators had begun to recognise a 'new free and easy sex-companionship'. Palling up was the thing, and meant that where possible men and women 'come together and form friendships . . . without any regard for the committal convention that marriage must be the object in view'.[22] Demographics and economics were also on the side of the lonely heart as serial dating and lengthy courtships were encouraged by both the cost of setting up a marital home during the prolonged post-war slump and the rising age of marriage. Wait before you weep became the new credo of the young and bright. From being a radical idea associated with eugenics, anarchism and the social networking experiments of do-gooders like W. T. Stead, the idea of some kind of formalised, pre-marital, adult friendship between the sexes had reached the mainstream. In spite of the difficulties faced by the lonely soldier, and the downfall of the *Link*, palling up was no longer merely an idea, or something that eager working-class adolescents did, but a practical possibility for grown-ups, thanks in no small part to the unfortunate Alfred Barrett – and an army of lonely soldiers. Faint moral qualms remained, however, and the potential dangers of advertising soon seemed to be all too evident.

Chapter Three

Peril in the Personals: Advertising and its Mysteries

When 31-year-old Irene Wilkins stepped off the train in Bournemouth on 22 December 1921, she thought she was about to meet a potential employer. In fact, she was about to meet her murderer. The daughter of a barrister who had died leaving the family in somewhat straitened circumstances, she lived with her mother in Streatham, south London, but she was a resourceful woman who had no qualms about going out into the world to make her way. She had served with honour in the Women's Auxiliary Army Corps during the war and, until a few weeks before her journey to Bournemouth, had been working in a boarding school. Now she was looking for another similar post and, having placed an ad in the 'Situations Wanted' column of the *Morning Post,* had come to Bournemouth in response to a telegram offering her an interview. The telegram, which was badly spelled, read as follows: 'Morning Post. Come immediately 4.30 train Waterloo. Bournemouth Central. Car will meet train. Expence no object'. It was signed 'Wood, Beech House'. Before setting out that day, Irene had wired back to say that she would catch that train and meet the car. What she was not to know was that a few hours later, her telegram would be returned to her home in Streatham – there was no such address as Beech House, and no such man as Mr Wood. The following morning,

Irene's body was found in some gorse bushes on the edge of the town. She had been killed by several blows to the head.

The police, led by Superintendent Garrett of the Bournemouth force, were stumped. Irene Wilkins knew nobody in the town or the surrounding area and there was therefore no way of conducting the usual hunt for clues among the victim's friends and acquaintances. There was no jealous lover or angry husband as there was in most murder cases. What could have been the motive? All that remained at the scene were the tyre tracks of a car. Had it been driven by the murderer? An impression of the tracks was duly made.

For several months, the police investigation made little progress. It was even suggested by the press that in their desperation they had turned to the assistance of local spiritualists who claimed to be able to contact Irene from beyond the grave. They offered the services of a 'sensitive' named Catherine Starkey, who was adept in the practice of psychometry, or soul reading. All that was required was something that had been touched by the murderer or the victim. On the basis of some matchsticks collected from the murder scene, Starkey claimed that the murderer was near at hand and that he lived in Bournemouth. She went on to give a detailed description of a man with a long, sallow face, big ears, high cheek bones, dark brown hair and hazel eyes. At one of her séances, Mrs Starkey channelled the spirit of Irene, and fell to the floor in what her followers claimed was the exact position in which the victim's body had been found.[1] Even with this proffered spirit guide, however, the police were not much the wiser.

Murders were much less common then, and were even

rarer in ultra-respectable Bournemouth, where the police could only recall two previous cases. As a result, Irene's fate attracted enormous attention, and in the fevered atmosphere of popular speculation that filled the vacuum of information, theories as to the murderer's motive were not slow to emerge. These vague ideas and half-truths reflected two ideas about the personal column which now appear exaggerated but which were stated over and over again at the beginning of the twentieth century: that it was by definition a space of mystery and concealment that could be understood only through a long course of familiarity with the scams and dangers which were hidden there; and that women were paradoxically both adept and vulnerable when it came to self-advertisement.

One self-appointed authority on the personal column, the police commissioner Sir Basil Thomson, who was fresh from directing the investigation of Alfred Barrett, suggested that the killer could well be a perverted seducer of the type he claimed to have encountered during the *Link* investigation, the kind who lurked behind the classifieds waiting to prey on vulnerable or adventurous women. The killer probably belonged, he said, 'to that class of persons who cannot live without sex adventure'. These were often men of leisure and wealth who would 'scan the columns of "sits required" in the hope of lighting upon one that promises this kind of adventure'. They were also men of a particular type, 'idle persons with time heavy on their hands', who would simply go off on a fresh quest if one attempted seduction failed. Generally, Thomson declared confidently, these men did not resent it when their victims resisted or turned them down, but in this case the element of violence suggested that the killer was a more brutal type. He was, Thomson suggested, likely to be 'of the mechanic class', probably a chauffeur.[2]

To add further drama to the case, there was speculation that white slavery might also be involved. Any advertiser or correspondent who went to the lengths that Irene's murderer had done to procure a victim must, it was assumed, be part of an international network of evil that lay concealed behind the classifieds.

> Lady cook (31) requires post in school; experience in school with 40 boarders; disengaged; salary £65 – Miss I. Wilkins.
>
> *Morning Post*, 22 December 1921

In spite of all the speculation, and the assistance of Irene from beyond the grave, the trail seemed to go cold. Then in March 1922 a sallow-looking man, named Thomas Allaway, not that different from the figure described by the Bournemouth spiritualists, was arrested for trying to impersonate his employer and to cash forged cheques. He was betrayed by his poor spelling, but bank staff soon decided that there was something remarkable about his handwriting, too. They were convinced they had seen the small, looping hand before – in the newspapers and at the cinema where the telegrams (complete with misspellings) and other evidence in the Wilkins case had been displayed on the screen before the main features.

Allaway, a chauffeur and a married ex-serviceman with a small daughter, was soon being questioned by the police in connection with Irene's death. In the course of their investigations they discovered a key at his lodgings which belonged to the lock of a garage where Allaway carefully hid his

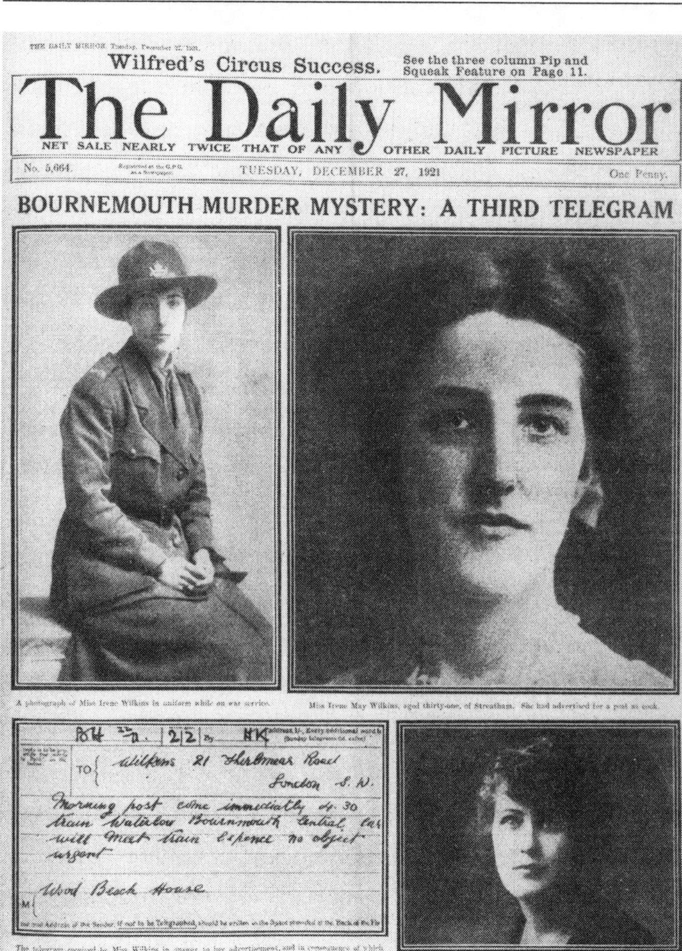

THE DAILY MIRROR Tuesday, December 27, 1921.

Wilfred's Circus Success.

See the three column Pip and Squeak Feature on Page 11.

The Daily Mirror

NET SALE NEARLY TWICE THAT OF ANY OTHER DAILY PICTURE NEWSPAPER

No. 5,664. TUESDAY, DECEMBER 27, 1921 One Penny.

BOURNEMOUTH MURDER MYSTERY: A THIRD TELEGRAM

A photograph of Miss Irene Wilkins in uniform while on war service.

Miss Irene May Wilkins, aged thirty-one, of Streatham. She had advertised for a post as cook.

TO { Wilkins 21 Hurlmear Road London S.W.

Morning post come immediately 4.30 train Waterloo Bournemouth Central car will meet train expence no object urgent

Wood Beech House

The telegram received by Miss Wilkins in answer to her advertisement, and in consequence of which she undertook the fatal journey. Detectives are anxious to trace messages in the same handwriting, and readers who can identify it are asked to communicate with the nearest police station.

Miss Betty Ditmansen received a mysterious telegram from Boscombe.

New interest is added to the unexplained death of Miss Irene Wilkins at Bournemouth on Thursday by the discovery of two other mysterious telegrams dispatched during the past two days from the Boscombe district. Both have many points of similarity with that reproduced above. The latest to come to the knowledge of the police was received by Miss Betty Ditmansen, of West Hampstead. Her suspicions were aroused, however, and she did not travel down to keep the appointment. (See news pages.)

War heroine Irene Wilkins and (below left) the fateful telegram that led to her death.

employer's car. It was an unusual one in the Bournemouth of the 1920s – a Mercedes – and when its tyre tread was compared with tracks found at the muder scene, it was found to match them. Allaway was duly charged with the murder of Irene Wilkins, though some doubts remained about whether he had acted alone and what his motive could have been. At his trial he remained impassive and impenetrable. On 18 August 1922 he confessed to the murder, and the following day he was hanged in the yard of Winchester prison.

It turned out that Allaway was, as Thomson had suggested, a man with time on his hands, and one who had actually spent his leisure hours searching for vulnerable women via the personal columns of the national press. Seven other women had received telegrams from Allaway making spurious job offers, but they had become suspicious after their telegrams were returned and had not travelled to the fateful meeting at the station. The fact that Allaway seemed to have established an elaborate system of entrapment encouraged ceaseless speculation about his motive. Why exactly had he attempted to lure women in this way? Had he been acting alone? Had he been the accomplice of some mysterious white-slaver or wealthy pervert?

This last suspicion remained strong even after Allaway had confessed to the murder. Many amateur detectives pictured him as an accomplice whose main role had been to drive the victim and her real killer from the station to the scene of the crime. The idea persisted, seemingly planted in the popular mind through the association of classified advertising with unseen, uncanny danger, that 'the crime was the work of some wealthy roué, sadist or blood maniac'. This was certainly the opinion of the Bournemouth spiritualists, who were supposedly told by the spirit of Irene that another man 'who has travelled much' was involved, and that 'someone else wanted her'.[3] A later theory, which fitted views of Allaway's class more closely, was that he had formulated some vague and indefinite plan for seducing some or all of the women he telegraphed. One writer, commenting on the case in 1927, pointed out that Allaway was being treated for syphilis at the time of the murder. In order to avoid the risk of being re-infected by prostitutes, he may have decided to direct his attentions, by force or otherwise, onto the respectable young women who advertised for situations.[4] The most plausible theory was that he had tried to seduce or rape Irene Wilkins who, drawing on the military training which taught her that a swift kick in the groin was the best way to deal with such men, had put up a spirited resistance. Allaway had then beaten her to the ground, panicked, and finally killed her with a tyre iron.

Women in Danger?

Irene Wilkins's murder was not the only one that year to link the mysterious personal column and the fate of young women. The most famous was the case of 'the French Bluebeard', Henri Desire Landru, who was convicted of killing seven women in Paris. Landru, whose enormous black beard, bald head and inscrutable manner gave him the appearance of a character from folklore, had spent seven years conducting a campaign of deception via the personals. He had contacted no fewer than 283 women through matrimonial ads, swindling some and supposedly luring others to their death at his isolated house on the edge of the city. He was finally and controversially convicted of killing some seven women in spite of the fact that their bodies were never found. The prosecution suggested that he had incinerated them in his domestic furnace, a claim given apparent credibility by his neighbours' recollections of thick, greasy black smoke emerging from his chimneys. The fact that there was no physical evidence allowed Landru to maintain his innocence with a series of implacable and constant denials, but these did not save him. He, like Allaway, was executed.

Gentleman, 35 years, income £400 yearly, wishes to meet really refined lady. Small income or capital would be preferred, but not absolutely essential. This is perfectly genuine; undeniable references supplied. No agents. View to matrimony.

The Times, 2 October 1915

Not surprisingly, the world of the small ad came under scrutiny again, just as it had during the *Link* trial. For many, these events simply confirmed a long-held popular belief about advertising – that it was the natural home of scams and frauds. Common Victorian dodges had included offers by quack doctors to treat sexual maladies or provide abortifacients, leading to a correspondence that soon turned into blackmail threats, while others ranged from money-lending schemes to employment agencies which required capital in advance, home-working scams and false trade directories.[5] The pervasive idea that all might not be quite right in the personal column provided inspiration for Conan Doyle's 1892 fictional investigation of *The Red Headed League*. Here a curious small ad asks for red-headed men to apply for a lucrative job which apparently involves no more than copying out the *Encyclopaedia Britannica*. In fact, as Sherlock Holmes and Dr Watson reveal, it is a ruse to cover up a daring robbery of the bank in the next-door office.[6]

But there was also a very contemporary social aspect to the fears that were expressed. In the immediate post-war period, concerns were continually voiced among more conservative commentators about the way the war had affected British society. It became almost a cliché that society was undergoing a kind of feminisation, a sort of creeping decay of moral fibre resulting from the war's erosion of older certainties and the evident fact that women like Irene Wilkins had taken on a whole new range of responsibilities to help bring about military victory. Although after 1918 many women who had worked in factories, hospitals or transport were forced out of their new roles by returning soldiers, their new feelings of self-assurance could not be erased – and the fact is that even after the war not only were more single women in employment than ever before, but they were also starting to make inroads into previously closed professions, such as the law and medicine. Conservative commentators worried about women's political rights as well, especially extending the vote to women over twenty-one in 1928, arguing that such liberalisation would create a frivolous 'flapper vote' which would be swayed by emotional appeals and good-looking candidates.

Refined spinster, age 23 years, height about five feet, Shop Assistant, considered a pretty brunette, Church of England, loving and vivacious; wishes to meet Londoner, 30 to 40.

Matchmaker, January 1928

Coupled with women's greater independence was a growing sexual assertiveness. Respectable women openly wore make-up, adopted androgynous flapper fashions with higher hemlines, cut their hair short and smoked in public. Naturally, Alfred Barrett's *Link* was one of the first papers to recognise and celebrate the fact that wartime had 'done for the girl today what ten slower years of evolution along natural and inevitable lines would have done for her'.[7] But this very independence had attendant physical dangers, as the fate of self-reliant Irene seemed to prove. Moreover, as the average age at which people got married crept ever upward in the 1920s, young, single women like Irene Wilkins were thought by many doctors and psychiatrists to be placing themselves in mental danger, too – susceptible to loneliness and all its attendant emotional difficulties. They were, in the view of one doctor, 'failures in love', who might easily fall into lesbianism, excessive masturbation, or even transitory and damaging love affairs in order to assuage their isolation.[8] They were also ready victims for the lures placed by predatory men via the small ad.

Many commentators seized on the classified ad as a way of exemplifying the tensions involved in this self-consciously modern femininity. They argued that the modern woman's new willingness to seek employment and adventure in the world made her particularly adept at the use of personal advertising – more so than most men. Because advertising of all kinds was thought to rely on an appeal to the emotions and unconscious desires, women were thought by many to be both good at self-advertisement and particularly susceptible to the charms of publicity. Women were not just claiming the full rights of citizenship, but were also thought to be the ideal, prototypical modern consumer.

The modern girl's new manner was, some argued, just another form of advertising. She was 'blatant' and 'conspicuous' and had learned the trick of artful self-presentation. The coded world of the small ad was therefore particularly suited to her talents. According to the *Daily Mirror*, commenting in 1919, women were better than men at writing ads: they understood the nuances of the words they used, particularly fashionable terms like jolly, unconventional, sporty and fed up, which at one level seemed perfectly respectable or 'refined' but, at another, offered hints of sexual availability. The *Mirror* argued that women advertisers had 'no ideas above "a good time", with "tall dark" – this is the favourite combination, it appears – "boys" who will take them out'. In the face of this female onslaught, the writer thanked heaven he was a man, and safely married.

In fact advertising and the 'modern' woman were regarded as interlinked manifestations of the contemporary world. As the protagonist of the satirical 1915 novel *Diary of a Flirt* put it, 'we live in an age of placards, and the person who wears most gracefully the biggest placard carries off the prize'.[9] The twentieth century was an 'age of advertisement', the *Daily Mirror* declared in 1922, which worked on the principle that 'if you don't advertise yourself nobody notices you'.[10] It was also noted that the coded language of the advert had begun to pervade ordinary speech. According to a 1928 satire, whereas talent in arms or speech had once been the hallmarks of the rounded individual, 'so now is the talent of advertisement', while everyday speech contained 'glib and pithy little catchwords' that mimicked the 'art of propagandism'.[11]

Men, however, were less sure of their place in this altered world. Those who had fought in the war, as Allaway had, were frequently assumed to have had their self-assertion and hence their masculinity compromised by brutalising and traumatic experiences. It became a cliché that men had either become callous, like Allaway (who had served with the transport corps), or emasculated by war neurosis, physical disability or simple fatigue. Damaged, disabled, impotent and just plain neurotic men filled the pages of post-war literature, from Lady Chatterley's wheelchair-bound husband Clifford to the suicidal Septimus who leaps to his death from the window of his psychiatrist's office in Virginia Woolf's *Mrs Dalloway* (1925). Ex-soldiers such as Robert Graves told of sleep disturbed by imaginary shells bursting on his bed, and walks marred by the faces of passers-by morphing into those of long-dead comrades.[12] All this contributed to a conscious feeling among British men of retreat from the heroic ideals which had led to the war, a turn towards the interior and the domestic.

The world of advertising, and of the personal column, seemed to reflect what the war had done to men. On the one hand, it became the natural territory of the callous, cunning or depraved seducer, just as Sir Basil Thomson had suggested. On the other, its very modernity and apparently confident sexuality bemused and intimidated many men. Some of the former type, men like the fraudster Edward Fitzgerald, who swindled women out of their savings in wartime Manchester, were said, like Henri Desire Landru, to be masters of the mysterious world of advertising, to possess 'in a remarkable degree the power of exciting the curiosity of women', and to have mastered the fine art of producing a compelling ad. Fitzgerald claimed that he was was 'good looking . . . not a "slacker"' and had a 'good income' which could be verified by 'genuine' references.[13] These were not atypical claims, and yet Fitzgerald was felt to be particularly adept at manipulating such stock phrases. Landru was similarly credited with being 'the most ingenious of advertisers', who knew 'that he has only to beckon and they [women] will surely follow'.[14] He was said to have had a 'half-hypnotic, half sixth sense which even the greatest criminologists and alienists of today have never been able to explain'.[15] He 'baited the trap with brilliance and with precision', posing 'always as something solid, respectable'.[16]

Other men, by contrast, were said to find the medium difficult to master. They couldn't cope with the frivolous or the insouciant. Instead they tended to be overly serious and old-fashioned. According to the *Daily Mirror*, they were 'much more in straightforward earnest than most of the women' and they were also disarmingly frank about their failings. One described himself as having 'been an ass', another was a '"common or garden" Tommy', another said he had 'no accomplishments', while others 'made no bones about being hard-up'.[17]

An investigation of the lonely hearts business by the muck-raking paper *John Bull* seemed at first to justify the concern felt by many for women advertisers in the harsh modern world of love and commerce. In 1927, the paper's celebrity columnist, Sydney Moseley, sought to expose the moral and physical dangers facing unsuspecting women by enrolling as a customer of several marriage bureaux, correspondence clubs and introduction agencies. Posing as a married sexual adventurer who could not obtain a divorce, he wrote to a matrimonial newspaper and agency named the *Matchmaker* and asked them to put him in touch with women seeking 'a good time'.[18] In spite of the fact that the *Matchmaker* claimed that all its advertisers were 'absolutely bona-fide and genuine' marriage candidates, his business was not refused, and on payment of ten guineas he was provided with a list of young female correspondents.[19] He then went through the same routine with three other clubs. One of these, the Universal Correspondence Club, he subsequently labelled as a 'sinister' and 'dangerous' operation.[20]

The proprietor of the *Matchmaker*, Thomas Owen, was duly denounced by *John Bull* for putting women in harm's way. He sued, but lost the case when it was revealed that for at least part of the time he was not, as he claimed, arranging marriages but fixing up what he called 'platonic friendships'.[21] One came from a 'businessman' seeking 'a young lady who would teach him dances'.[22] Another was from a 'Lady . . . stylish in dress' who wanted 'a real good pal' to 'come and have a cup of tea'. Several others clearly specified 'companionship' rather than marriage. As for the non-sexual friendships that several ads claimed to be seeking, they did seem to set out the characteristics of the desired partner in suspicious detail.[23] The judge doubted whether true 'platonic friendships' between the sexes could actually exist, and questioned the motives of those seeking such relationships. The word platonic was, he said, little more than a euphemism to 'cover up what, on the face of it, any man or woman of the world must see is calculated to lead to illicit moral relations being established'.[24]

One young woman, identified in court only as 'Miss X', who advertised with the *Matchmaker*, and who was the key defence witness, made it clear that this picture of danger and seduction was all wrong, and that women like her were perfectly able to look after themselves. They could, she said, easily spot the danger in people like Landru or Fitzgerald, and they had not been defrauded, as *John Bull* claimed. Modern women, she said, were perfectly able to use and understand the various codes and conventions of the medium.

> Bachelor, age 23, height 5ft 4in, medium complexion, well built and strong, sailor on submarine, just won competition for good looks, wonderful eyes, wishes to meet a young girl, 21 to 23.
>
> *Matchmaker*, quoted in *The Times*, 22 May 1928

Miss X, who had used the 'platonic branch' of the *Matchmaker* to find 'man pals', vigorously defended her right to do so. Through its good offices she had become, in her words, 'fixed up', or 'practically engaged' to a respectable soldier. In contrast, *John Bull*'s barrister Norman Birkett tried to portray Miss X as a representative of modern womanhood and all its problems. 'I am going to suggest to you', he said, 'that you are the kind of girl who ought to have somebody to save you from yourself in this kind of thing.'[25] He reminded her that she was only nineteen at the time of her first advertisement, and that she 'might have been ruined by some ruffian or adventurer'.[26] Miss X, however, vehemently disagreed with this suggestion. In her view, she did not need saving at all, was 'quite capable of looking after [herself]',[27] and regarded Birkett's alarmist scenario of ruin and disaster as highly unlikely. She also rejected his claim that she was 'on the brink of a very great tragedy', pointing out that the four men she had met via the *Matchmaker* had not been drunken immoralists or racially alarming Mexican 'half castes', as *John Bull* claimed, but 'very nice and quite proper persons to be introduced to her'. She had had 'no alarming experiences and was not the victim of fleecing, unscrupulous or otherwise'.[28]

Undeterred by the unflappable Miss X, *John Bull* continued to investigate companionship ads and correspondence clubs throughout the 1920s, but also continued to find advertisers who were perfectly at ease with what they were doing and open about the social opportunities they felt the world of the small ad opened up for them. They could see the danger in unscrupulous men who said they merely wanted a partner for a 'hotel divorce', or who suggested experimenting with drugs. Even after setbacks like these, such women retained their sense of adventure. One of the members of the Universal Correspondence Club, for example, said that she joined because she was 'sporty [and] fond of life'. Another became a member because she liked 'anything with a bit of adventure attached'. The story of Miss X also had a happy ending, at least according to the *Matchmaker*, which shortly after the trial proudly and repeatedly announced her marriage to 'Mr J.P.A.D.', the man who was supposed to have placed her in so much peril.[29]

Although women continued to argue that they were quite at home in the anonymous world of the personals, the ads still fascinated and intrigued. In the 1930s, for example, George

Orwell argued that papers devoted to classified ads, such as *Exchange and Mart* or the *Matrimonial Times*, minutely reflected their readers' interests and could therefore be seen to operate as a sort of guide to the mysteries of the collective unconscious.[30] But the suspicion they aroused would not go away. In the wake of the *Link*, Allaway and Landru cases, moral campaigners across Europe continued to argue that this world of coded language must be hiding all sorts of wickedness and concerted criminality.

Chapter Four

White Slavery by Post

As 19-year-old Kitty Weston was walking along the London–Brighton road on the night of 9 September 1925, a car drove past. She dropped her suitcase into a ditch and ran into the undergrowth, terrified that it was her employer, Hayley Morriss, come to take her back to his strange and lonely house on the edge of Ashdown Forest in Sussex. It turned out, however, to be a policeman who had come out to search for her. Once he had tracked Kitty down, she was taken back to the safety of the police station in the nearby town of Uckfield.

Earlier that night, Kitty had thrown her belongings together and taken off on foot, trying to put as much distance as she could between her and Morriss's home at Pippingford Park. She had only started work for the former Shanghai stockbroker two days before, but had swiftly found that things were not quite how she had expected them to be. True, there were certain attractions to the new job: discipline was not particularly onerous, nor were the tasks handed out by her employer and his young housekeeper, Madeleine Roberts. It did seem rather surprising, though, that dancing, parties and trips to hotels and clubs in nearby Brighton were also included. Moreover, Morriss's attitude to his collection of young, pretty housemaids was, to put it mildly, more than merely affectionate.

Kitty's brush with the man later to be dubbed by the papers the 'Shanghai Millionaire' began when she answered an advertisement in *The Times* of 31 August 1925: 'Young girl of gentle birth required to look after large dogs in the country. Live in. Experience unnecessary. Common sense essential'.[1] Kitty, being fond of dogs and anxious to escape her domineering stepmother, replied to the ad and was summoned to an address in Jermyn Street. There, she met a pretty 21-year-old named Madeleine Roberts, who said she was Morriss's ward and who offered Kitty the job at £1 per week. Kitty arrived at Pippingford Park on 7 September, and at first all seemed normal. The job was undemanding, consisting mainly of feeding the Irish wolf-hounds which Morriss kept for breeding. The following day, however, Kitty discovered that Morriss did not treat his domestic staff in the same way as most other employers did. That afternoon, while he, Kitty and Madeleine chatted in the drawing room, Madeleine put a record on and Morriss insisted on dancing with his new kennel-maid. 'You are going to come to my room tonight,' Morriss said, all the while holding Kitty just a bit too close. She resisted, at which point Morriss said, rather ominously, 'Little birds that won't sing must be made to sing.' Madeleine Roberts's reaction was simply to smile: she had clearly seen it all before.[2]

Young girl of gentle birth required to look after large dogs in the country. Live in. Experience unnecessary. Common sense essential.
The Times, 31 August 1925

That night, Morriss came to Kitty's room wearing only his pyjamas. He sat on the edge of her bed before reaching out and holding her so tightly she could hardly move. Claiming that she seemed to be freezing cold, he suggested getting into bed with her. When she refused, he left, saying that he knew when he wasn't wanted. Soon afterwards, in a complete panic, Kitty phoned a friend in London who alerted the local police. They found her later that night wandering with her suitcase by the road.

On the surface, Morriss, a 33-year-old bachelor, seemed perfectly respectable, if slightly unconventional. Originally from Sussex, he had spent much of his life abroad and, in the course of working as a stockbroker in Shanghai, had amassed a huge fortune. He returned to Britain shortly after the First World War and took up a leisurely country-house life, entertaining his society and sporting friends with shooting, dancing and bathing parties. But, as the police swiftly discovered, it was not just Kitty Weston who had been the object of his advances. Six other girls, ranging in age from 15 to 20, who had worked at Pippingford in the previous year were found to have been recruited in a similar way, and then given the same regime: light duties, dancing and bathing parties, suggestive conversation and attempted seduction. One was Bessie, a 14-year-old parlour maid. She had told another member of staff in 1924 that she wanted to move from the room next door to her employer and, when asked why, replied, more in exasperation than fear, that 'Mr Morriss comes into my bedroom every night and I am absolutely fed up with it. Hang it all I'm only fourteen and he might leave me alone sometimes.'[3] Another was a 17-year-old maid who recalled long conversations with Morriss about the facts of life, during which he boasted that he had never 'done in' any girls because he knew all about contraception, his favoured methods being the douche or the quinine pessary.[4]

The way in which Morriss went about recruiting new staff followed a fairly similar pattern each time, and relied extensively on classified ads and domestic agencies. The ads for kennel-maids were placed by a 20-year-old woman whose real name was Ellen Ferguson, but who styled herself as the glamorous Russian Patricia Alexeieva, known simply as Pat, and who had first encountered Morriss when she worked as a waitress at a Lyons Corner House restaurant in London. She also interviewed some of the girls at a flat in London to see if they met Morriss's requirements in terms of class and looks. Madeleine Roberts played a similar role. She was not Morriss's ward, as she had told Kitty, nor even his housekeeper, but his mistress, having originally come to Pippingford as a cook in 1923. Both women helped to recruit local girls by registering with various domestic agencies in Tunbridge Wells and Brighton. They also helped Morriss to lure young shop assistants or working girls he happened to encounter on his travels. Some were found at dance halls and one was propositioned by Morriss while she was serving at Hamley's toy shop in Regent Street in London and offered a weekend at Pippingford. Morriss and Roberts also used to cruise around Brighton in a Rolls-Royce, offering suitable-looking candidates a drive in the country. On one of these jaunts, Morriss had looked one girl up and down before telling Roberts not to engage her as she didn't 'look clean'.[5] Two women who later gave statements to the police did go for a drive out to Pippingford and were offered the usual jobs looking after the dogs, but they refused anything more. It seems that Morriss, with Roberts's help, forced himself on several teenage girls. His mistress was even alleged to have procured her own 15-year-old sister for her employer's teenage harem, a charge later dropped. Locals claimed, probably exaggeratedly, that as many as 100 girls had been to the house in the past few years, none of them staying very long.

About a month after the discovery of Kitty Weston in her roadside hiding place, Morriss and Roberts were charged on twenty-two separate counts, mainly of procuring girls under the age of 21, and indecently assaulting one of the teenage maids. Morriss was also charged with having sex with one of his 15-year-old domestics. Even though all the girls except one had ostensibly given their consent to Morriss's advances, evidence that he had procured under-age girls seemed clear, plentiful and damning. Passing judgement, Mr Justice Avory told him that he was guilty of 'pursuing a systematic course of procuring young girls and young women' for the purpose of gratifying his 'loathsome lust upon them'.[6] Morriss was accordingly sentenced to three years in prison, while Roberts received nine months. Hard labour was attached to each sentence.

In their comments on the case, the press emphasised what they felt to be a peculiarly oriental aspect to the whole affair. The elements of sadism were said to be characteristically Chinese, no doubt picked up by Morriss during his long years in the East. The number of girls who came and went at Pippingford summoned up images of a desert sheik gathering a harem about him. Pippingford itself seemed a very un-English place; it even housed a menagerie of exotic animals and birds, including storks and wombats. Morriss was, the *News of the World* decided, 'A Sultan in Sussex', a

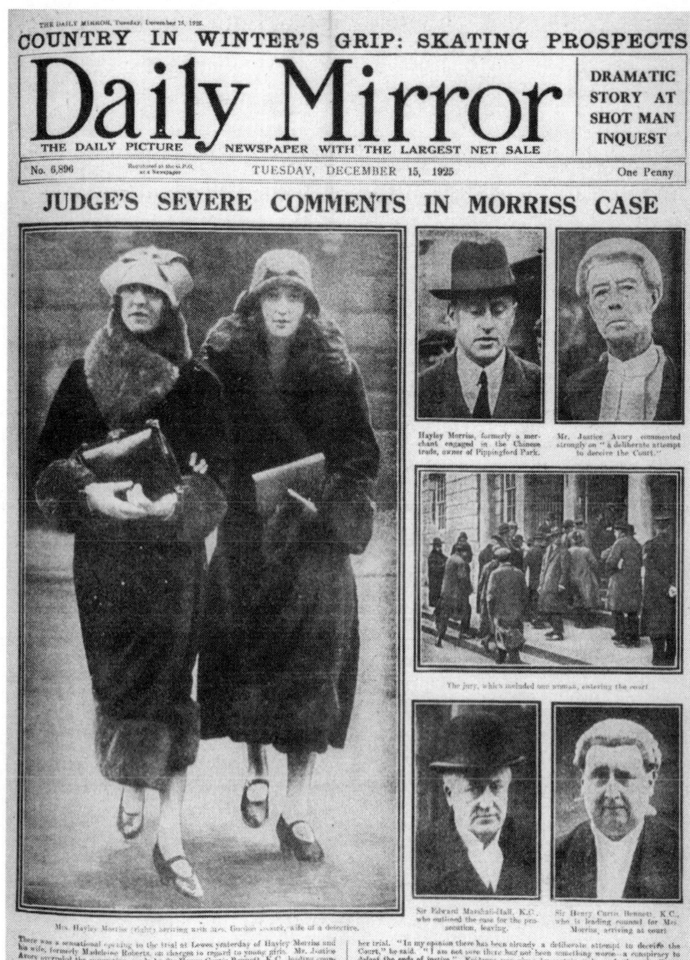

THE DAILY MIRROR, Tuesday, December 15, 1925.

COUNTRY IN WINTER'S GRIP: SKATING PROSPECTS

Daily Mirror

THE DAILY PICTURE NEWSPAPER WITH THE LARGEST NET SALE

DRAMATIC STORY AT SHOT MAN INQUEST

No. 6,896 — Registered at the G.P.O. as a Newspaper — TUESDAY, DECEMBER 15, 1925 — One Penny

JUDGE'S SEVERE COMMENTS IN MORRISS CASE

Mrs. Hayley Morriss (right) arriving with Mrs. Gordon [illegible], wife of a detective.

Hayley Morriss, formerly a merchant engaged in the Chinese trade, owner of Pippingford Park.

Mr. Justice Avory commented strongly on "a deliberate attempt to deceive the Court."

The jury, which included one woman, entering the court

Sir Edward Marshall-Hall, K.C., who outlined the case for the prosecution, leaving.

Sir Henry Curtis Bennett, K.C., who is leading counsel for Mrs. Morriss, arriving at court

There was a sensational opening to the trial at Lewes yesterday of Hayley Morriss and his wife, formerly Madeleine Roberts, on charges in regard to young girls. Mr. Justice Avory overruled the suggestion, made by Sir Henry Curtis Bennett, K.C., leading counsel for Mrs. Morriss, that he should hear medical evidence regarding her fitness to stand her trial. "In my opinion there has been already a deliberate attempt to deceive the Court," he said. "I am not sure there has not been something worse—a conspiracy to defeat the ends of justice." Evidence was given by certain girls, and when the Court rose the Judge ordered that both Mr. and Mrs. Morriss be kept in custody.

Madeleine Roberts (main photograph, on right), with an unidentified friend, and Hayley Morriss (top, second from right) outside the Court in Lewes where they were tried for procuring under-age girls.

'man from the East, about whom the only thing English is his colour'.[7]

The case seemed to show that every dark fantasy about classified advertising had been proved true. Morriss also seemed to fit almost exactly the profile of the white-slaver conjured up by moral campaigners and the tabloid press in their campaigns against immorality of all kinds. Just like the figures of white slavery legend identified by the press, Morriss had clearly operated a system of entrapment through classified columns and employment agencies, his wealth seemed to insulate him from conventional morality, and like some figure of folklore, he lived in an isolated mansion in a dark forest. White slavery, or something very like it, appeared to be only too real.

Investigating White Slavery

Was white slavery – the idea that there was a network of international prostitution – merely a myth? Was Morriss an actual white-slaver, or did he just fit the mythical template? It is obvious from observing our own world that disparities of wealth do create a supply of sex workers, and that these women are then moved across international frontiers as part of the migration of all kinds of labour. Often, prostitution is most apparent at the boundary between rich and poor, and many enter sex work because of the unenviable choices which poverty presents. Prostitution in the late nineteenth century resulted from extreme disparities of wealth, just as it does in the present. However, the lurid legends of international white slavery were, more often than not, used to obscure rather than illuminate this reality. Instead, when they weren't being used to attack immigration – and to try and prevent an imagined horde of foreign and especially Jewish prostitutes from coming to Britain – they were used by the press to encourage a much broader sense of moral unease about the modern woman.

> Are you Lonely? Why not join the Progress Club for correspondents, unconventional friendships, educational progress, and less lonely life. Members everywhere. Write for information.
>
> *T. P.'s Weekly*, 22 September 1911

The origins of the belief in white slavery stretch back to the 1880s and the efforts of moral campaigners to eradicate prostitution by raising the age of consent and implementing harsher penalties for procuring. To back their efforts, groups like the National Vigilance Association (NVA) began to circulate sensational tales of women being abducted or lured from Britain to work in brothels in Belgium, France or even Argentina. All these white slavery stories tended to share certain melodramatic features: a young innocent girl, often a virgin, unwittingly decoyed into prostitution by a cynical older woman like Madeleine Roberts; an evil seducer – often an older, aristocratic pervert, not unlike Hayley Morriss. The young innocent would be taken away from her home and promised employment just as Kitty Weston had been. She would then be drugged or be forced to submit to sexual slavery.

The most famous white slavery scandal of the Victorian period – and the template for those that followed – occurred in 1885 when the editor (and later inventor of the social network) W. T. Stead set out to prove that it was possible to buy a pre-pubescent virgin openly on the streets of London. Through the offices of an ex-prostitute turned moral campaigner called Rebecca Jarrett, he found a 13-year-old girl called Eliza Armstrong, for whom he paid £5. For Stead, the story, which he ran at great length in his paper the *Pall Mall Gazette*, had mythical implications – it was no less than the 'Maiden Tribute of Modern Babylon', a modern transposition of the legend of the minotaur who consumed young virgins presented to him for sacrifice in his labyrinth. Stead splashed the story across his paper for weeks on end, seemingly proving that white slavery existed at the heart of the Empire. But something was not quite right. Stead claimed that his intermediary had bought the girl from her parents, who knew exactly the kind of trade into which she was being sold. However, the girl's mother, Mrs Armstrong, came forward with a different version of events. According to her, Jarrett had offered to take Eliza into domestic service, a proposition to which she had readily assented. In the end, the police took the Armstrongs' side, proceedings were taken against Stead for abduction, and he served a short term in prison. For the rest of his life, on his birthday, he would put on his prison uniform, just to remind himself how virtue could be misunderstood.[8]

Like many sensational tales of seduction, the Maiden Tribute affair showed up the problems of the white slavery stories. For all Stead's sound and fury, and the undeniable existence of prostitution, it was never proved that you could actually buy a young virgin. Nor could it be proved that some widespread system of organised international white slavery really existed. However, the belief that women were in danger from white-slavers did gain powerful adherents, and in 1902 sixteen European governments agreed to implement an International Convention for the Suppression of White Slave Traffic.[9] The signatories agreed to arrange for observers to monitor railway stations and ports in order to detect those involved in the white slave trade. Foreign prostitutes were to be questioned about their origins and the way they had been 'recruited'. In England a 'White Slave Traffic Branch' was set up at New Scotland Yard and fifty workers were employed to meet young unaccompanied women at major ports and rail terminals in London. The idea that foreign – especially Jewish – prostitutes were flooding London's streets led in part to the passing of the 1905 Aliens Act, which sought to restrict immigration from eastern Europe.

Between 1909 and 1912, sections of the press whipped up a huge white slavery panic, mounting a 'Great Crusade' against the traffic in a 'National Campaign of Grave Importance'.[10] Classifieds were also identified for the first time as the key method of the white-slaver. The press described announcements which appeared to be offering domestic situations, theatrical work or companionship, but which masked brothels and prostitution rackets. Typical of the media coverage was a story run by the popular weekly *MAP, Mainly About People* in 1910. It described how an alleged 'Professor' had serially advertised for 'a young Christian lady, who may be poor, with a view to marriage'. He had then seduced and blackmailed his many victims. The paper went on to warn women about the dangers lurking in advertisements seeking girls to join musical or dancing parties for continental tours, and others for women's employment agencies, artists' models and companionship. It concluded that such advertisements were 'only a small part in the organized campaign' of white slavery.[11] It was partly due to this constant press coverage that in 1912 new criminal justice legislation, nicknamed the 'White Slave Act', was passed by parliament. It sought to protect young women by tightening the laws against sex below the age of consent (16) and providing for new penalties – including whipping – for those procuring women for the sex trade.

In fact, prostitution as a whole was actually in decline in both legend and in fact, as the numbers of prostitutes in Britain began a long-term fall from the Edwardian period onwards. By 1913, the police were beginning to conclude that trying to control prostitution by monitoring ads, watching massage and manicure parlours and interviewing foreign streetwalkers was a fruitless task. The White Slave Traffic Branch at Scotland Yard had found little evidence that a widespread and organised sex trade across international frontiers actually existed. White slavery panic was, it seemed, the product of hysteria, and had, the CID concluded, 'been aroused by a number of alarming statements made by religious, social and other workers, who spread the belief that there was a highly organised gang of "White Slave Traffickers" with agents in every part of the civilised world, kidnapping and otherwise carrying off women and girls from their homes to lead them to their ruin in foreign lands'. Every single case of alleged abduction, drugging or false advertising which had been investigated had proved to be false.[12] Moreover, when the NVA established a service which provided for its officials to meet and offer assistance to unaccompanied young women arriving in London by train, they found that the vast majority refused to have anything to do with them.

> Professor, 42 years old, with money, wishes to make the acquaintance of a Christian young lady, who may be poor, with a view to marriage.
>
> *MAP, Mainly about People*, 12 February 1910

But if the white slavery panic was on the wane before 1914, it started to re-establish itself both during and after the First World War, as worries grew about what were felt to be increasingly lax moral standards in contemporary society. A new group of women was identified – women who were happy to be taken out on dates, might well be sexually available, but who were seeking amusement rather than payment. The names conjured up for them told of their marginal moral status: they were 'amateurs' or 'charity girls'. It was feared that they could all too easily find themselves lured into actual prostitution. By the 1920s, some moral campaigners in Britain had become sceptical about the more lurid tales of white slavery that had characterised the Edwardian period, but for others including the NVA, the Morriss case was a vindication of their beliefs.

These suspicions were also still shared on an international scale, as trans-national bodies continued to look for evidence of white slavery, convinced that there were sinister, organised forces behind prostitution. In 1927, the League of Nations' report on white slavery concluded that 'the international Traffic in women is still an ugly reality', and that it 'continues to defy the efforts to suppress it made both by Governments and voluntary agencies'.[13] Classified advertisements continued to be scanned for evidence of the codes that, if cracked, would show the extent of prostitution, not to mention other forms of sexual depravity. In 1927, Dr Ninck, the Swiss delegate to the Seventh Congress on the Traffic in Women, revealed that in the previous five years, 10 per cent of all Swiss cases of prostitution had been 'directly connected' with newspaper advertisements. In a further 30 per cent 'some advertisement or other [had] played a part'. Ninck identified various common categories of advertisement, along with certain phrases and euphemisms that undoubtedly cloaked 'immoral or perverse intercourse'. These included matrimonial ads which seemed to reduce the holy state to a 'business transaction', apparently innocent 'Requests for money or loans', such as that from 'Two smart, blonde young ladies' who sought help with a 'momentary financial difficulty', and friendship ads in which 'we must often suspect homosexual inclinations and intentions'. Ads for midwives, he suggested, were also suspect, often being placed by maternity homes offering secret abortions.[14]

In Britain, popular culture took up the white slavery story where some moral campaigners and most government agencies were now leaving off, and exposés appeared at regular intervals in the press and popular fiction. A classic example is *The Story of a Terrible Life* (1928), a history of the life and work of a notorious white-slaver and brothel madam written by the veteran pressman Basil Tozer. It went through seven editions in as many years and was followed by an equally lurid sequel. According to Tozer, no fewer than 15,000 women went missing every year in Britain, and 5,000 disappeared from London alone. They had probably disappeared into the maw of white slavery. The questions were how had it happened, and who was behind it?

The answers came from 'Madame Messaline', a veteran madam and procurer whom Tozer had met in a military brothel in France during the First World War, and who was happy to reveal a whole range of tricks she employed to lure unsuspecting young women to their doom. Her repertoire included a network of bogus artists' studios seemingly populated by sincere and innocuous-looking young men, the manufacture of her very own brand of drug which rendered girls dreamy and listless, and the recruitment of an army of bachelors intent on seduction. These men, Messaline's 'cadets', were hired to seduce women into white slavery and were recruited through cunning and subtle advertising. The ads generally mimicked the format of companionship, announcing a 'lady of artistic temperament' who wished to correspond with a 'young man similarly interested', or a 'well-placed, elderly gentleman' after 'friendly intercourse with a young man'. Perverts of all kinds were alerted by sly references to 'Lesbos' or 'Masoch'. Many of those who replied were insufficiently worldly or glamorous and were therefore unsuitable to Messaline's evil purposes. These innocents were turned away, but those who knew the secrets of the personal column anticipated that things were not as they seemed. A substantial proportion of respondents, Messaline said, answered the ads 'knowing well that they will be wanted for something not quite – well, you know'.[15] Her men were instructed to hang around places where young working girls congregated, to gain their trust, and finally to introduce them to their 'aunt', who would initiate the women into the world of prostitution.

Friendship clubs and correspondence circles were equally useful to the white-slaver, Messaline claimed. She was amazed that the police let these organisations continue without harassment. Messaline knew of many in her own line of business who had established 'friendship-forming circles' which 'I have reason to know, generally means – well, you can guess what it means'. These clubs, like the *Link* or *T. P.'s Weekly*, claimed that they were helping the countless lonely men and women in the world and as such sounded 'very nice and human and philanthropic', but were in fact exactly the reverse. Tozer himself set out to investigate, and later claimed to have unmasked the 'X.Y. Bureau' friendship club as a front for part of Messaline's evil network.[16]

> Friendships can be formed immediately through the U.C.C, an up-to-date genuine and reputable introductory medium with over 10,000 members both at home and abroad. All classes suited, either sex. Established over twenty years. Suitable introductions are guaranteed.
>
> Quoted in *John Bull*, 30 April 1927

Even the dullest of Tozer's readers ought to have been able to tell that his narrative was somewhat exaggerated. His claim, for example, that 15,000 women went missing each year was based on a fairly deliberate misinterpretation of NVA figures. Fifteen thousand was actually an inflated estimate of the total number of single women met by the NVA's officials at railway stations and ports in the period before the war.[17] Even the League of Nations estimated that numbers involved in international prostitution were in the low hundreds, not the high thousands. Tozer's books do, however, tell us much about contemporary morals and moral concerns. They were an attack on the free and easy modern spirit which might lead women into illicit sex or even worse. As one reviewer put it, the *Story of a Terrible Life* was a timely warning to 'foolish young girls who think that because someone is "nice" they must therefore be "safe".'[18]

The Morriss case gave a final fresh impetus, and much promising new material, to these cautionary tales. By the time Tozer's book appeared, Morriss had already been convicted, and on what looked like clear evidence. On the face of it, Tozer's tales therefore had more than a ring of truth about them. But was the Morriss case as straightforward as it seemed? He was certainly unappealing, even wicked, but the more troubling question for those who attacked him was whether modern girls were in fact complicit in their own downfall, agents in their own seduction.

Morriss, for all his efforts to get his staff into bed, was clearly offering an implicit bargain, and one which some of the women involved, especially his acolytes Patricia Alexeieva and Madeleine Roberts, were only too willing to accept. While they and several others were over the age of consent, others, such as the three 15-year-olds who Morriss was charged with corrupting, were, in the circumstances, much less able to exercise any independence of mind. Morriss's wealth made it difficult for young, poor and unworldly women to resist. His relationship with his mistress Madeleine Roberts seems to have bordered on the abusive, and it was reported that they were often seen having terrible arguments. Coming from a poor and perhaps criminal background, Roberts had clearly found it difficult to repel all Morriss's blandishments and was said to be strongly 'under his influence'. Pat also remained true to Morriss to the end, refusing to give evidence against her patron, and remaining in attendance throughout the trial, having installed herself in a Brighton hotel.

Moreover, in spite of everything, Morriss was a popular employer, as even the press conceded. One of his advertisements attracted 300 applicants, and his servants, although not handsomely paid, lived in a style that other domestics would have envied. One of the strangest things about the case, the *News of the World* noted, was that Morriss got 'as many [servants] as he liked – when other folk could not obtain domestics for clean and decent homes'. Part of the reason for this was that 'they had a good time, as most of them confess'. Morriss's favourites were dressed in fine clothes; they were 'unstinted in luxuries and taken about in a big car to all the gay functions of the neighbourhood'. All the servants 'enjoyed independence that would have staggered the ordinary domestic', and were 'at liberty to order anything they wanted' with Morriss footing the bill.[19] At the trial, one 15-year-old maid admitted that she had been 'perfectly happy' at Pippingford Park, while another 17-year-old 'of good education' said that 'Morriss was perfectly kind and courteous to her', and had 'made no attempt to force her to do anything she did not want to do'.[20] Some of his domestics certainly objected to him, not least Kitty Weston, but not all of them did, and he seems to have been

> Lonely Friends – Correspondents, companions secured through the Modern League. Sections: story-collectors, holiday in common, bachelor's guild; lessons exchanged; hobbies – stamp svp – Secretary.
>
> *T. P.'s Weekly*, 5 May 1911

popular locally. Police inquiries revealed two local girls – 'the talk of the village as being very fast' – who had stayed with Morriss and who telephoned him regularly.[21]

This testimony raised troubling questions about what adolescent girls – especially those above the age of consent – could know and do. But the case rested in part on a legal contradiction in which the backgrounds and motivations of the various women in the case were central. According to the Criminal Law Amendment Act of 1885, under which Morriss was charged and which was passed in the climate of hysteria that followed the Maiden Tribute case, procuring women between the ages of sixteen and twenty-one for sex was only a crime if the girls involved were not 'common prostitutes or of known immoral character'.[22] In other words, 'good' girls were protected by law, but 'bad' girls had to look after themselves, whether they had consented to sex or not. The 'Shanghai Millionaire's' status was therefore ambiguous: he had certainly cajoled women into sleeping with him, but could he be a white-slaver if many of his victims were not actually innocent? The whole case showed the limits of white slavery stories as a way of comprehending contemporary life. They just did not fit the complications raised by cases like this and were rapidly lampooned into obsolescence by writers like Evelyn Waugh.

Morriss did not go quietly, and he spent the next few years suing the press over alleged inaccuracies in their reporting of his trial and complaining loudly about infringements of prison rules. He even acquired supporters. An MP who introduced a bill to increase the penalties for men like Morriss noted with incredulity that a correspondent had compared the Sultan of

Sussex to a 'Christian Martyr', arguing that Morriss had been unjustly convicted in the face of widespread evidence that the girls had more or less consented to his advances.

The small ad, though, remained in the dock. The extent to which it was involved in white slavery – indeed the very existence of white slavery itself – might now be in question, but moral campaigners still felt the personal column might be the home of 'fast' women and unsavoury men. Prostitution, it was argued, was funded by the trade in pornography, and the idea that pornography could be found lurking everywhere in the pages of the personal columns was not perhaps as far-fetched as it seems.

Chapter Five

'Bits of Fun': The Lost World of Pornography and Fetish

In December 1922 an Exeter bookseller named Cyril Benbow placed a series of advertisements in several of the illustrated papers that had pioneered the companionship ad. The first one read, quite simply: 'Books: Gentleman has collection of Books for sale. State requirements and enclose SAE'. It looked pretty innocuous, but since advertising managers of the time were only too aware that even such bland announcements could be used to mask something rather unsalubrious, Benbow was obliged to confirm that he was exactly who he claimed to be – a bona fide bookseller. He accordingly told the *World's Pictorial News* that 'the books in question consist of those . . . by such well known authors as Voltaire, de Musset, Tolstoi [and] E[ugene] Sue', and stated specifically that he was *not* offering 'erotic or other objectionable stuff'.[1]

He was, however, being rather economical with the truth. From his office on the quayside in Exeter he had often imported erotica and pornography from its centres of production in Paris, Barcelona and Vienna for sale in Britain. He would then send out speculative circulars to potential customers, at first sending lists of respectable books, and then, by a series of hints and leading questions in further correspondence, would try and find out whether they wanted anything stronger. If they did, he would then send them a full list of pornographic material. For 10s and 6d you could read all about *How Milliners Amuse Themselves.* For 15s a dozen, you could order postcards of 'beautiful white backsides', 'young ladies pregnant' or 'splendid women with enormous breasts', not to mention views of various other body parts and pictures depicting various sexual acts. Nudes draped suggestively in diaphanous fabrics were half that price. More expensive 'high-class' material, which had been the staple of the erotic book trade since the late Victorian period, was also on offer – books such as *White Slaves* (7s and 6d), *Pendula Venus, The Girl Astride*, or *Flossie, a Venus of Fifteen* (all 25s). Benbow's range of stock even extended to dildoes, 'male and female'.

Benbow was certainly not alone in the porn business. Many other individual dealers and agents utilised the classified columns of the British and imperial press to capitalise on a vast demand for pornography, erotica and all kinds of other material. One measure of the size of the industry is the sheer amount of material that was declared obscene. Whereas in the late nineteenth century the pornography business had been measured by the tonnage of print seized by the police, by 1938, individual magazine titles were targeted, 400 of which were outlawed – the most hard-core of which were estimated to have circulations in excess of 100,000 copies.[2] By 1951 more than 65,000 similar magazines, 28,000 photographs and 11,000 postcards were being seized and destroyed annually by the police, numbers that represent only a fraction of what was actually in circulation.[3] This clandestine business was, for many social commentators, a sign of a deep sickness in European society. Those with a conservative agenda argued that pornography was a sign of moral corruption that should be stamped out at all costs. More liberal or left-wing commentators declared that official censorship prevented honest discussion of the reality of sex in British society, and had thereby created a generation of sexually repressed people who could only find an outlet in the cheap and nasty products of a man like Cyril Benbow. However, despite police confiscations and social disapproval, the trade nevertheless continued to grow.

Benbow's working methods illustrate the way in which the industry operated in the first half of the twentieth century. Essentially, he found new customers via advertising, and he also cooperated with agents throughout the country who distributed his catalogues and books on commission. One of his key contacts was a London dealer named Mervyn Hyde, who had first been drawn to Benbow's catalogue by its selection of fetish photographs. His first purchases were of photos and books about 'high heels, tight lacing, discipline, heel drill, etc etc, including Female Impersonation', about which he was 'ardently enthusiastic, not only in theory, but also in practice'.[4] Hyde clearly hoped that in Benbow he had found someone who shared his interest in restrictive corseting and high heels, but Benbow demurred, and their relationship remained strictly at the level of business. According to Hyde, who made contacts and money by selling and exchanging customer lists with other agents and dealers, there were 'many gentleman of the nobility, the gentry and the better class of commercial and industrial men who long for these goods without any idea of where they can get them'.[5] Thanks to Benbow and a carefully assembled network of producers, dealers and agents brought together via the classifieds, he was able to satisfy his customers' needs.

Hyde had actually been in the porn trade since the 1890s when he claimed to have done an 'enormous business', selling up to £50 worth of books at a time to various regular customers via adverts in risqué bachelor papers – weeklies with innocently cheeky titles like *Photo-Bits, Illustrated Bits, Bits of Fun* and *Pick Me Up*. As befitted his profession, he was a past master of decoding classified ads.[6] He would pore over them endlessly, scrutinising them for particular signs or tell-tale words. If he thought he had found something promising, he would write to the box number listed and carefully sound the person out. If all went well at this stage, he would then send catalogues of naughty postcards, literary erotica and fetish material. Hyde's diary lists various ads and box numbers from the national and illustrated press. He was, for example, inevitably alerted by the word 'Corsets' at the beginning of an ad that appeared in *The Sunday Times* in August 1922, noting that the correspondent was offering to put him in touch with 'a lady of good social position' who wanted to 'correspond with others interested in tight lacing'. Elsewhere in his diary, he listed names and box numbers from the illustrated weekly *Fun*, the *Daily Mirror* and the *Evening News*, along with another from *The Times* placed by 'Wasp Waist', seeking any 'lady or corsetiere' with experience and interest in 'the super-corseted figure'. He made notes to remind himself about the preferences

Rare Books, Art Magazines, etc ENGLISH AND FOREIGN. Special low price offer for French Illustrated Magazines and Periodicals, 1/-, 1/6-, 2/- each post free. Retail lists sent with orders.

Business Chances, September–October 1936

of his customers and advertisers, from the Herefordshire vicar who liked 'all kinds of stuff, lots of it', to a woman in Slough ('dildoes'), and another in Oxford Circus who always took 'high class stuff'.[7] Hyde also noted the addresses of a Bristol shoemaker who could provide 'very high heels', and a shop where 'hair killer' could be bought in order to help with the drag act that was Hyde's other occupation. A 'social circle' with similar interests could also be found meeting in Lancaster Gate in West London. From this huge variety of people, shops and ads, Hyde built up a list of over 100 contacts and customers.

As well as having links to an embryonic fetish community in London, Benbow and Hyde developed contacts with the producers of porn on the continent. The kingpin of European pornography in the early twentieth century, and the main supplier of hard-core material to the British market was Ricardo Gennert of Barcelona, aka V. Fleury, aka Leonard Sucr, a man well known to the police, and who had long been involved in selling obscene books in Britain. Little is known about Gennert, except that he began to appear in police reports in the 1880s, and that he operated through a series of aliases and addresses in Paris, Barcelona and Vienna. Benbow first encountered this pornographic mastermind via a small ad placed by Gennert in the *Times of India*. His initial enquiry was an ordinary business one, but he soon found himself being encouraged to become one of Gennert's English agents for his catalogue of literary erotica. At first he refused, worried about the risks involved, but when Gennert told him that his cut of this lucrative trade would be 33 per cent, he changed his mind.[8] All went well for about a year until the

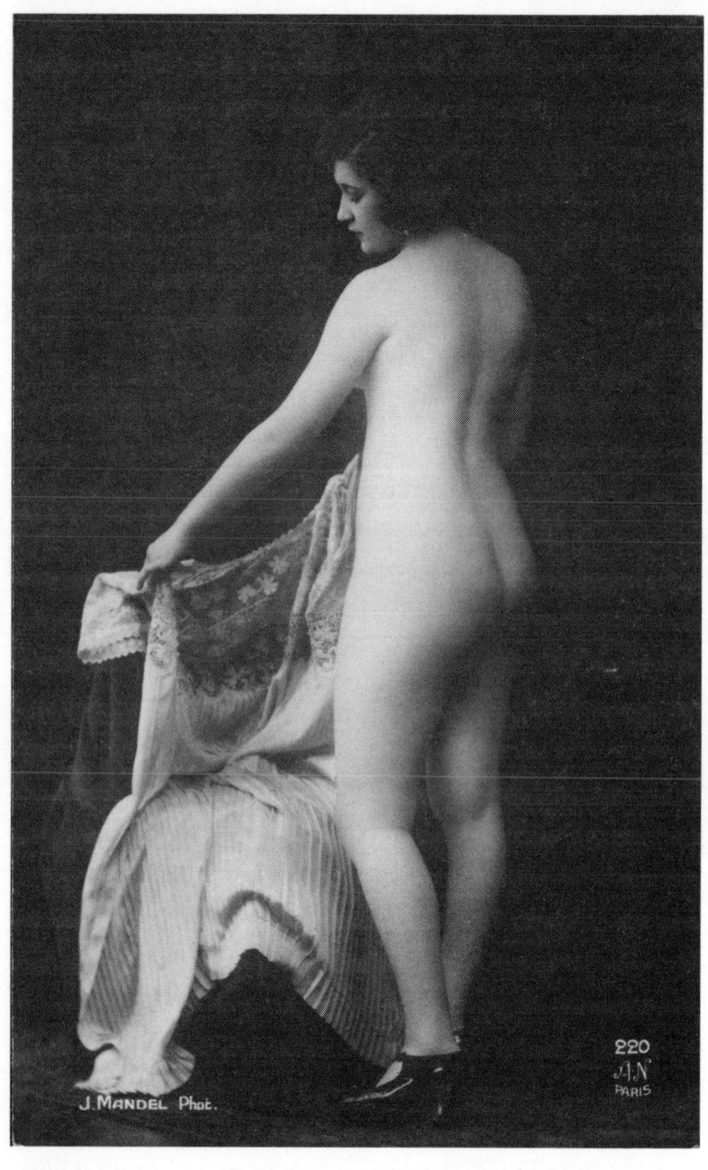

Erotic postcards such as this (produced in Paris in the 1920s) were the stock-in-trade of many British dealers between the wars.

police raided Benbow's office. He and Hyde were tried and convicted of conspiring with Gennert to corrupt public morals and publish obscene books. Both were fined and sentenced to a short prison term.

Pornography vs the Police

Police action against Benbow and Hyde may have closed down one conduit for illegal material, but it had no discernible effect on the wider market in erotica, pornography and fetish material, and although the authorities engaged in a protracted war of manoeuvre against obscenity, the legal barriers they created never came close to defeating the dealers. The first anti-obscenity statute was the Obscene Publications Act of 1857 which outlawed material that was deemed to have the power to 'deprave and corrupt'. Then there was a series of laws passed in the 1880s regulating the mail and empowering the Post Office and Customs to seize and open suspect packages.[9] 'Indecent Advertising' was banned in 1889. This particular law was then extended twice, first in 1911 to cover birth control products and circulars, and again in 1917 to cover quack remedies for VD. By the 1920s, whole warehouses of books were being labelled obscene, including such classics of modernism as James Joyce's *Ulysses*, D. H. Lawrence's *Lady Chatterley's Lover*, and *The Well of Loneliness* by Radclyffe Hall. By 1909 the police were claiming to have suppressed much of Britain's domestic porn production, but this somewhat exaggerated claim concealed the movement of pornography production to the continent, where it was sent to Britain through carefully constructed mail-order networks, which were themselves dependent on cleverly worded classified ads.[10]

As pornography became an international trade, governments across the continent began to see the necessity of co-ordinating their efforts against it, and a series of international conventions against obscene publications was drawn up as part of the wider assault on the elusive white slave traffic. As Basil Tozer's story of the legendary white-slaver Madame Messaline showed, vigilance groups thought that there was an umbilical link between the traffic in women and the sale of obscene publications. Tozer's semi-fictional white-slaver Madame Messaline, for example, was supposed to cultivate a refined taste in literary erotica and scientific books about sex, while her agents were assumed to peddle vast quantities of erotic postcards as one way of getting clients in the mood. However, the international conventions against obscenity did not produce any significant action against the porn business, and were soon little more than bits of paper. Pornographers remained just as elusive as the semi-mythical white-slavers.

The supply of erotica and pornography was sufficiently varied to satisfy just about any taste, and appealed to everyone from the customers of backstreet shops to respectable suburban householders buying through the mail. By the 1920s the main constituent of the market was the thousands of American and French pulp magazines, with titles like *Wild Cherries*, *Silk Stocking Parade* or *Paris Nights*, mostly featuring 'saucy stories', or topless women dressed in black stockings. Equally numerous were postcards of nudes, available either airbrushed, or, more daring, 'unretouched' (showing pubic hair), and also coy 'art studies' of the naked form. Amateur writers of erotica provided mimeographed manuscripts containing unbelievable tales of sexual athleticism. Worst of the whole lot, at least in the opinion of the Home Office, were the flagellation magazines known as 'Hollywood' stories after their titles – *Hollywood Revels*, *Hollywood Nights*, *Hollywood Tales*. By the mid-1930s it was claimed that ten million pulps a month were sold in America alone, while other pulp titles and Hollywood-type mags sold in their hundreds of thousands across the British Empire.[11]

> Sell Sex Books. A big Dollar Seller. Sample 50c and list of other big sellers included . . . Dixie Mail Service Box 67, King North Carolina, USA.
>
> *Business Chances*, December–January 1935–36

To talk of a 'porn industry' before the mid-1960s is a bit misleading. Despite the quantities sold, pornography was something of a cottage industry, involving numerous individual dealers like Benbow and Hyde, many of whom had other jobs and who dealt in erotica as a sideline. One major Soho agent of the 1930s was also a wine salesman, while another twice-convicted Birmingham dealer in 'Art Studies' was a grocer, his partner an electrician.[12] Larger-scale publishers and organised crime only really moved in after the mid-1960s when mainstream magazines such as *Penthouse* started to make large profits. Gangsters then began to take over the porn trade and concentrate it in the West End of London, particularly Soho. Before then, profits were too small and the risks too great to attract such large-scale operations, and pornography distribution was shared by towns and cities like Folkstone, Exeter or Watford, all of which would have at the very least one mail-order dealer like Cyril Benbow. Rather as at present, when the internet and the wide availability of video has encouraged 'amateur' pornography, so in the 1920s and 30s a popular vogue for writing and the increasing availability of cheap cameras helped create a non-professional world of sexual fantasy. People wrote their own stories and sent them in to the pulps, they took photos of their wives (and sometimes husbands), they exchanged photos, and sold porn back to its producers when collections became embarrassingly large. All of this activity was hidden, or semi-hidden, at the back of mainstream papers, in *Exchange and Mart*, the *Times of India*, or the pages of adventure pulps.

Porn dealers – amateur and professional – had to be adept at evading the law. Book dealers had swiftly realised when the 1857 Act was passed that while their shops and printing presses might be vulnerable to seizure by law, selling pornography by mail was not yet an offence. This realisation ushered in an era of euphemistic adverts aimed at what were called 'private readers' placed in such papers as the *Sporting Times* and the *Favourite* which aimed squarely at young men. The Post Office Acts of the 1880s meant that one now had to be careful how material was circulated, but the sheer volume of mail made it impossible for the authorities to spot every package containing obscene literature circulating in Britain or coming from abroad. At the beginning of the twentieth century, erotica would arrive from France hidden underneath copies of the French newspaper *Le Matin*, 'real hot photos' would be posted through a series of forwarding addresses to throw the police off the trail, and sealed containers would be sent to 'highly respectable' women employed as intermediaries and dealers. Police crackdowns did close down some

British pornographers temporarily, but they tended simply to move their business to Paris, from where they sent direct mail to their key market among army officers, university students and others in single-sex institutions. One common trick of the Edwardian dealer was to pose as a private individual who had just inherited a mysterious box containing 'private books and such like', which he was prepared to offer at a bargain price. In one such case, two tons of erotica sent to Britain from the Continent were seized.[13]

Other similar ruses were employed by the sellers of contraception and rubber goods in order to get round the law against indecent advertising. Public advertising of birth control was made illegal in 1889, and the law was tightened again in 1911 to redefine what was 'public' in more expansive terms. Manufacturers of contraceptive devices prevented from advertising openly tended therefore, from the late-Victorian period onwards, to send unsolicited circulars to a wide variety of people of all classes, from noblemen to labourers.[14] Leading local figures such as doctors or businessmen were often singled out as key recipients. A common tactic of rubber-goods salesmen was to study the births columns of the local press and then to send circulars to the new parents which praised the benefits of small families and advertised condoms, pessaries, sponges and books on birth control. Before it was outlawed in 1911, other kinds of display were common. In Birmingham in 1906, a sandwich man patrolled the streets, extolling the virtues of Newton's, 'the Best and Cheapest Medical, Surgical and Rubber Appliances' on a placard three feet wide.[15]

The cheap and saucy weeklies that thrived just before and after the First World War, and that were known collectively as the 'illustrated press', helped cater to the tastes of those whose interests inclined towards pornography and fetishes. Titles such as *London Life*, *Illustrated Bits*, *Photo Bits*, *Pick Me Up*, and a series based repetitively around the idea of fun, such as *Fun*, *Film Fun*, *Photo Fun*, *New Fun*, *Bits of Fun* and others ad infinitum, shared a basic formula: naughty-but-nice illustrations and gently satirical cartoons. Comic strips shared column space with sporting and theatrical gossip, pictures of chorus girls and film stars in skimpy stage wear, alongside vaguely indecent reproductions of 'classic art', the latter being a useful excuse to depict the naked female form – even if it was only a smudgy copy of a distantly remembered Old Master. Short stories dealt with contemporary moral dilemmas, such as the pressing question: 'Can Modern Flappers Love?' (the answer being yes, women in this male imagination invariably being game for anything), or investigated the phenomenon of the companionship ad with a piece examining the possibility of 'Husbands on the Hire System'.[16] *London Life*'s favourite women were young, resourceful, modern and fashionable, just like the 'low-necked, short-skirted misses one sees in the streets', who were 'thoroughly respectable, hardworking girls', perhaps a little 'hoydenish', but 'certainly not either indecent or immoral'.[17]

Illustrated papers also had a more obviously perverse side that was apparent in their correspondence columns. These were regularly colonised by S&M advocates and fetishists like Mervyn Hyde, and were often filled with intense speculation on topics that ranged from restrictive corseting, bondage and high heels, to detailed meditations on the merits of bathing fully dressed, being a 'human pony' (wearing a bridle and reins), one-legged girls, transvestism and new women's sports like wrestling, often given by Madeleine Ferguson, 'The famous lady athlete, physical Culturist and wrestling referee'.[18] Although these subjects contained fetishistic and queer themes, they remained veiled in euphemism, and as they did not discuss actual sex in an explicit fashion, they flew below the radar of official concern and legal censorship. Fetish correspondence, though suggestive, could always claim some kind of alibi and rely on its readers for a double meaning.

The roots of such fetish correspondence, which outlined in detail the various methods and pleasures of constriction, reached back into the nineteenth century, when anonymous fetishists made a practice of taking over the pages of fashion periodicals like *Modern Society* (1883–98) or the *Gentlewoman* (1893) and household magazines like the *Family Doctor* (1886–93). Discussion of S&M could and did continue for years in this way, providing an important channel of communication between fetishists. One of Benbow and Hyde's specialist lines featured collections of this correspondence, amounting to over 60,000 words and including the Victorian fetish bibles *Corset and Crinoline* and *Figure Training*.[19] When the correspondence in these magazines became too strange, or when the editor finally began to object, the fetishists moved on to another journal. At various times, all illustrated weeklies, but especially *London Life* and *Fun*, played host to the writers of fetish correspondence.

That said, the overwhelming tone of papers like *London Life* was not so much perverse as worldly: the average reader was clearly encouraged to view himself as an insouciant bachelor and man about town who didn't take life, or sex, that seriously. In other words, this was the world of bohemian-yet-refined masculinity that Alfred Barrett's *Link* espoused, and it is no surprise to find the *Link* and many other correspondence and lonely-hearts-type clubs being advertised, written about or imitated in these papers. The reader of *Fun* or *London Life* could join a correspondence club, or, like 'WGB', find a girlfriend via the 'Do You Want a Pal?' companionship column. He, at least, was satisfied with the results of reading these bachelor papers, and wrote to *London Life* in 1921 to express thanks for being put in touch with so many girls, the result of which was that he had 'met one of the young ladies [and] . . . she is much better than I expected to find'.[20] Similarly, readers could buy pornography or erotica via an advertisement from one of the mail-order companies, and purchase contraceptives from the same source. These papers were not only naughty but nice, they could also provide practical access to cultures of illicit sex.

Chic Photos, 72 Unique Subjects and list 2d to adults only. Splendid Sample Collection, 2s.
London Life, 15 January 1921

In spite of its tolerant and good-humoured ethos, the illustrated press certainly had many enemies. These unconventional readers, the enthusiastic customers of small-time book dealers and contraceptive salesmen, were thought by some to be in terrible danger, mainly from themselves. To those on the right, pornography and indecency were a certain sign of moral decay, while to those on the left, they signified widespread sexual repression. As the socialist sexual reformer Alec Craig put in 1937, those who bought pornography and sought fantasy were outcasts from normal society, people 'unable to satisfy their sexual desires in the world of reality, by reason of misfortune, ignorance, lack of enterprise, or inability to effect the necessary modifications and compromises'. They were the people who had given up struggling with desire in order to seek satisfaction in a world of unreality. Porn was a sign of sexual repression in both society and the individual, and a substitute for real emotion. It could only be removed by extensive social reform, 'rational sex education' and 'the creation of social conditions which will obviate sex frustration'.[21] But were the customers of men like Benbow and Hyde really such tortured or immoral individuals? For many readers, there turned out to be much more to 'private reading' than simple gratification.

Chapter Six

Mail Order: A Dirty Education

In 1942 the sleepy country town of Bodmin in Cornwall briefly achieved notoriety as the national capital of mail-order obscenity. This somewhat dubious distinction came about when police paid a visit to a local company, the Economy Educator Service, and discovered that its range of stock extended considerably beyond the sort of books that a business with such an unassuming name might be expected to sell. Trial and conviction for its owners duly followed.

The Economy Educator Service – motto, 'The Man Who Reads is the Man Who Leads' – had been set up in 1925 by a farmer named Ralph Clemoes and his wife Lillian. In the early days, it focused on self-help literature – books on boosting one's confidence, success in business, and correspondence courses on shorthand. Then in 1933, as the enterprise boomed, a list of what were called 'sex books' was added, along with a 'confidential advice bureau' dealing with 'sexual difficulties'. The sex list was carefully advertised in the press and publicised via countless circulars posted indiscriminately to addresses across the country. The range of titles on offer was impressively wide, including 'Famous Books on THE BODY BEAUTIFUL, NUDISM AND SEXOLOGY that you have always wanted to have' and titles that could not be obtained elsewhere 'at any price'. Another company circular advertised the erudite and comprehensive *Encyclopaedia of Sex Practice*, edited by the eminent sexologist Norman Haire, by asking the reader: 'Will You Pay the Penalty for Ignorance?' The rest of the list included ninety-one titles on sexology alone, as well as major works on birth control, sexual technique and sexual history, nudism (including Sensible Sunbathing, 'a practical guide for nudism'), the pseudo-lesbian photo collection *The Well of Loveliness*, as well as a scholarly series on the history and practice of flagellation. All were available either to buy or to rent at a reduced price with an option to buy. At the moment when the Clemoes were finally arrested for sending obscene articles through the post, Economy Educator was doing well and employed fourteen staff.[1]

Why had the Clemoes, with their relatively innocent, even mainstream list of books, been singled out for prosecution? The problem lay mainly with the ambiguities of the law against obscenity, which made indiscriminate advertising of sexual material especially suspect. While the content of any obscene article was important in law, and in general, themes like full-frontal photographic nudity, as well as sadomasochism, homosexuality and other 'deviations', made prosecution more likely, it was also true that in practice, laws against obscenity focused mainly on the assumed audience of any obscene article. This interpretation dated back to the 1857 Obscene Publications Act and an 1868 court ruling on that Act which stated that the test of obscenity was whether any publication had the potential to 'deprave and corrupt'. The courts usually interpreted this to mean that obscenity was proved if any publication could be said to have fallen into the hands of those – mainly assumed to be the young, women, or those not educated enough to tell the difference between science, literature and pornography – who might be 'depraved and corrupted' by reading it. Deciding whether a book or picture dealing with sexual matters was legally obscene was therefore largely dependent on an estimation of who might see it. Obscenity didn't just depend on who the audience was, though, but also on where you were. Outside London, many serious works of sexology which had gone unmolested in the capital were prosecuted because local, and especially northern, magistrates felt that provincial readers were much less sophisticated, and might therefore be reading a serious work for entirely the wrong reasons.

In retrospect, it is hardly surprising that the Clemoes fell foul of this law, since although most of what they sold was not legally obscene, their output did contain more daring items. It was, for example, not illegal to show the naked human form in their nudist or 'art' series, provided that pubic hair was not on view and the body was not posed 'suggestively'.[2] However, like many literary and photographic depictions of sex and nudity at the time, some of the Economy Educator's output was artfully and precariously posed on a legal borderline. By selling and, more importantly, advertising, books which celebrated

Birth Control 1929 Illustrated Treatise Free, By a Well Known London Physician. An up to date Comprehensive 1929 Treatise containing most valuable information for the married. Worth pounds, and should be in the hands of all married people. Send post free to all mentioning this paper together with catalogue of PRO RACE appliances fully explaining best and safest methods to adopt.

London Life, 6 July 1929

flagellation, such as John Swain's scholarly *Pleasures of the Torture Chamber* and Cooper's Victorian classic *A History of the Rod in All Countries*, as well as endless series of 'art studies' and photographic nudes, the Economy Educator placed itself in ambiguous legal territory. The line was crossed, in the opinion of the police, when Economy Educator inevitably sent some of its thousands of circulars to decidedly the wrong people. One such person was a Mrs Whitaker of Exmouth in Devon, a respectable middle-aged lady who on 16 April 1940 wrote to the National Vigilance Association complaining that she had recently been inundated with unsolicited circulars from Economy Educator. She had, she said, absolutely no interest in nudism or flagellation, and wondered if anything could be done to stop this kind of indecent publicity. In response, Frederick Sempkins, the Secretary of the NVA, said this was the second complaint he had received in a week, and that he knew of several members of the NVA who had received similar circulars. He forwarded the complaint to the Home Office and the wheels of justice began to turn.

Advertising Obscenity

Part of the reason for the authorities' interest in the Economy Educator's pamphlets was the fact that the mail was full of such material in the 1930s and 1940s. Norman Haire's *Encyclopaedia*, for example, one of the Clemoes' bestselling books, was advertised by its publishers in 1935 via the distribution of 250,000 leaflets. These were sent, they claimed, to 'various classes of official and professional persons whose names were selected from directories'. Haire's book was educative, certainly not prurient, but the reason it was prosecuted lay in the way in which it was advertised, especially in the indiscriminate publication of leaflets suggesting something racier than mere science. Serious books on sex were legally acceptable if they were clearly being bought by serious, intelligent people who could be trusted to know the difference between information and titillation – who would, in other words, not be 'depraved and corrupted' by reading about sex. The fact that many serious books on sexual reproduction and anatomy tended to be quite expensive also generally exempted them from legal persecution as a high price supposedly put them out of the reach of unsuitable purchasers. However, advertising via small ads and circulars brought such works within the ambit of the 'wrong' sort of curious reader, attracted, according to the magistrate trying the case against Haire's advertisers, by a 'preliminary account of certain subjects emphasized by capital letters'. Most seriously, the same magistrate ruled that the circular he was scrutinising was clearly framed in such a way as 'to increase the sale of the book by attracting the attention of the public whose interest in the subject was very far from being scientific'.[3] Even Haire himself admitted that the circular, with its invitingly capitalised sections and sensational promises, had been 'in bad taste'.[4] Indiscriminate advertising was deemed to be worse than the books themselves, and both Haire's case and that of the Clemoes ended in conviction for the Economy Educator and Haire's advertisers, Amalgamated Publicity Services.

As these cases showed, the Obscene Publications Act was a relatively blunt instrument that led to a series of legal judgments based on estimations of a hypothetical audience. Even serious books, therefore, tended to be nervously published, in small print-runs and at a high price to ensure that only the right people, such as doctors or barristers, would be counted as their intended audience. When, in 1927, the writer Walter Gallichan wanted to buy the highly academic *Frigidity in Women* by the German sexologist Wilhelm Stekel, he found that the only way he could do so was to claim that he was buying the book for a doctor, and he even had to produce a letter from the doctor in question, confirming that this was the case.[5] It was not surprising, therefore, that even serious books on sex sometimes fell foul of the courts. These included Haire's *Encyclopaedia* (prosecuted successfully in 1935 and again in 1950), Edward Charles' investigation of sexual biology, *The Sexual Impulse* (successfully prosecuted in 1935) and Eustace Chesser's bestselling general guide, *Love Without Fear* (unsuccessfully prosecuted in 1942).

If buying such books openly was fraught with difficulties, borrowing them from public libraries was often not much easier. They tended to practise a form of self-censorship, rarely stocking books on subjects such as birth control. Potentially problematic books, such as Richard Aldington's war memoir *Death of a Hero* (1928), which dealt mildly with soldiers' swearing and sexual preoccupations, often ended up being locked away or hidden behind the counter. To borrow them required a potentially humiliating encounter with a librarian. Those books that did escape censorship and become popular classics, like Marie Stopes' birth control series *Married Love* (1918) and *Enduring Love* (1922), which were scandalous to many readers simply by virtue of being about sex, had to stick rigidly to the conventional morality of monogamous marriage and to avoid explicit description of any actual sexual acts. By the 1940s even these *successes de scandale* were starting to look old-fashioned and reticent.[6]

Given how difficult it was to buy serious books on sexual matters openly, or even to borrow them, it is scarcely surprising that mail order should have become such an important channel for their distribution. Nor is it surprising, given mail order's relatively tight profit margins and fear of prosecution, that some companies were not particularly discriminating about what they sold. The many small-time mail-order operators and rubber-goods stores which populated this market therefore began to sell an eclectic mixture of mainly imported texts, some pornographic, some literary, and some scientific or anthropological, advertised in personal columns and box ads in *London Life* or mail-order trade papers like *Business Chances*. Ads placed in 1921 by the chemist C. F. (later L. L. Charles), of Tottenham (established in 1887), for example, offered erotica like *Paris by Night*, *All About Girls* or 'Chic Photos, 72 Unique Subjects', but they also listed instructive works on birth control such as *Knowledge a Young Wife Should Have*, at 2s and 6d, and *Family Limitation* by the renowned American birth-control guru Margaret Sanger, the latter thrown in free with each order.[7] In addition, this family business sold condoms and other contraceptives by post. Similarly other major advertisers of the 1930s and 40s, including Seymour's Surgical Stores of the

Birth Control. Approved Surgical Rubber Goods. Trade list and samples 1s (Returnable).

Business Chances, June–July 1935

Strand, Hygienic Stores (many branches in London), W. George of Leicester Square, General Supply Stores of Weymouth, and Beatall of Merthyr in South Wales, tended to sell a mixture of birth control and sex books. Other small-time advertisers appealed to the same elevated and intellectual taste by presenting 'Artists and Connoisseurs' with 'Beautiful Life Camera Studies . . . Rare Books, Magazines, English and Foreign, Artistic Cine Films'.[8] Even American dealers, such as the Panurge Press of New York, who promised 'the surprise of your life', and who advertised in the back of widely available American humour pulps like *Ballyhoo*, sold by mail order a wide variety of high-sounding 'oriental love books . . . sophisticated sexualia, esoteric anthropology' alongside less intellectual 'erotic adventures'.[9] This kind of unsupervised and eclectic reading alarmed the authorities, which concluded in 1936 that perhaps the chief danger of the pulps was not the pictures of naked women which appeared in them, but 'the list of advertisements which some of them contain, and which might well be in many cases but a cloak for debasing and immoral activities of many kinds'.[10] Certain stock phrases, such as those that promised books for 'private readers' were clearly designed to signal to the potential purchaser the true nature of what was on offer.[11] Seeing these phrases, readers learned, as one customer later admitted, to expect 'books similar to those sold in France and dealing with sex in a fairly outspoken way'.[12] Similarly, 'Advanced Studies' of the human form advertised in the West Midlands in 1927 indicated to one Shropshire farmer that he might anticipate postcards of what he politely called the 'Roman statuesque figure variety – something denoting

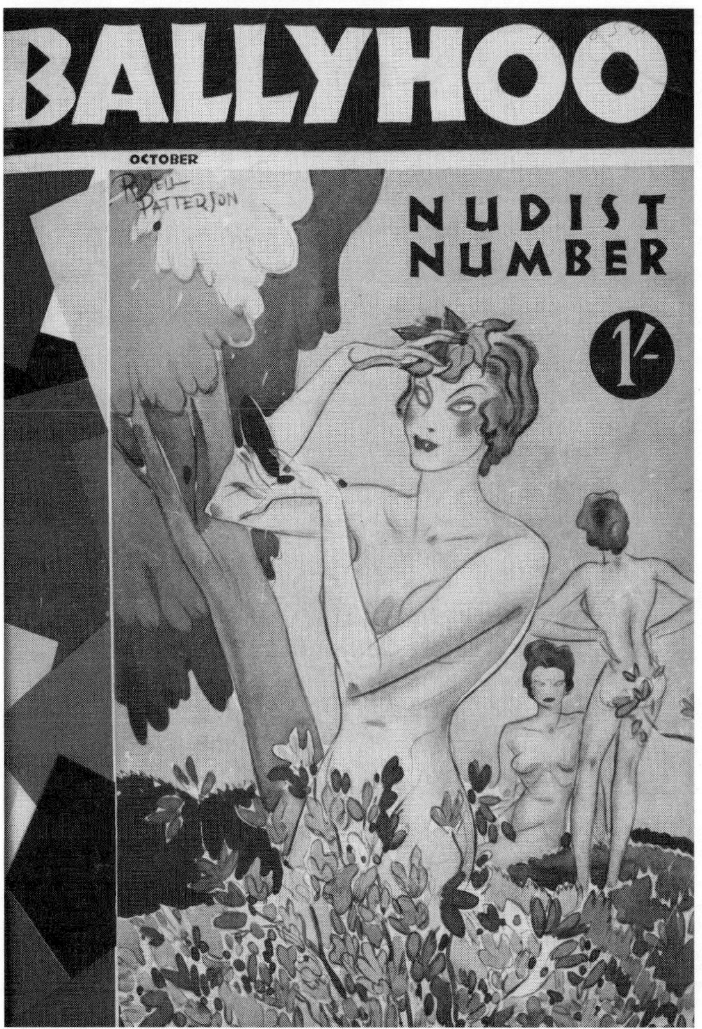

The October 1933 cover of the American humour pulp magazine Ballyhoo *– one of many in the 1930s and 1940s to include the ads of book dealers.*

strength and health.'[13] Advertising of this nature, which was a constant feature at the back of French and American pulp magazines, persisted for some years after the end of the Second World War, ensuring that the pornographic and the scientific were sold side by side.

The various companies involved in selling material of a sexual nature reflected the eclectic nature of the market by flattering their readers' belief that they were not merely thrill-seekers, but were also on a quest for self-improvement. General Supply of Weymouth affirmed that their list of nudist titles, sex histories and birth control guides were not for just anyone, but for the discerning man of the world. Their output, they claimed, comprised '*Intellectual Books for Intelligent Readers* by reputable publishers (not popular rubbish)'. Such companies promoted an intellectual-practical approach to sex which stressed that it was a vital part of self-improvement in general. Southern Mail Order, which operated from a residential address in the staid seaside town of Bognor Regis, offered a broad range of popular sexual psychology and pseudo-pornography, but it also promoted courses on self-improvement ('How to be Taller in 12 Days'), advice on money-making, and books on how to raise livestock. Direct Book Supply of Kingsbury in North London, a company that advertised in the classified columns of the literary monthly the *Writer*, offered a similar range. Like the Economy Educator, it was both a library (lending out its list for a small price) and an ordinary mail-order outlet. It presented its readers with nine categories of educational and pornographic books for 'PERSONAL use of members of Professions, Psychologists, Social Workers, Students of Psychology and responsible adults, for the purpose of serious study'. From its catalogue, one could choose anthropological classics on South Sea islanders by Malinowski, scientific studies by the greats of sexology like Krafft-Ebing or Stekel, pseudo-historical works like *The Harem* ('A huge fully illustrated volume of novel interest . . . Contents include Harem customs, Punishments, Eunuchs . . . etc etc.'), or straightforward erotica: 'High Heeled Yvonne by John Bagley . . . A very extraordinary novel of intense interest to lovers of the bizarre in female embellishments, with a background of Parisian nightlife, many aspects of glamour and luxury, sordidness and sex are treated in absorbing detail. Very strictly for adults only'. The more expensive of these titles, 'rare books . . . practically unobtainable at any price', were also the most pornographic.[14]

Although individual mail-order companies like these were essentially small-time operations, collectively they offered education of a haphazard kind to men, and sometimes women, wanting to understand sexual matters. They also represented a particular sexual ethos, which cleverly encouraged and flattered a masculine desire for competence. In the 1930s and 40s it was, after all, a man's job to know about sex. For a woman to have this sort of knowledge was to go against ideals of femininity and to run the risk of being branded 'fast'. That's not to say that women in the 1930s did not know about sex, or even to suggest that they were not customers

---

Important. The Enclosed Matter Refers to a subject of great interest to all married people, namely, contraception. If you have no desire for information on this subject, it is requested that you destroy this packet unopened.

Circular distributed in Reading, 1931

---

of mail-order libraries or porn dealers (the dealer Mervyn Hyde's diaries contain several women's names), but it was clearly important not to show that you knew too much. The historian Kate Fisher has shown, through a series of interviews with men and women who married in the 1930s, that sexual knowledge and understanding of matters like contraception (whether using artificial methods like condoms or 'natural' techniques like coitus interruptus) was assumed to be the man's, not the woman's, responsibility. The blend of pornography and sex education retailed by mail-order libraries, rubber-goods shops or book dealers served this masculine need for competence and knowledge. It helped readers to be men who were 'in the know', reading and leading in the way promised by Economy Educator.[15]

The files of a police investigation into one of these mail-order dealers tells us quite a lot about the sort of customers they attracted. Park Trading, a mail-order operation and shop based in Notting Hill in West London, was one of the more successful mail-order services of the 1940s, and like so many others sold everything from straightforward pornography to academic studies, taking in on the way 'unretouched' photographs, home-made 'sex stories' in mimeographed manuscript, psychoanalytic case histories masquerading as porn, sex instruction books, eugenic primers, and the frankly erotic works of the American literary novelist Henry Miller (not published legitimately in Britain until 1963). When the police raided the company, they seized its address book and, as usual on these occasions, then went to interview the company's customers. They turned out to represent a cross-section of society from company directors to farm workers, via hotel managers, electrical engineers, shop assistants, schoolboys and bank clerks; even policemen and Scottish aristocrats were patrons. Their varied backgrounds showed that Park Trading and its competitors were able to reach right into the suburban home and into the heart of middle-class respectability. Few customers fell obviously into the category of 'perverts'. The police described one typical customer as a respectable, even intellectual sort, 'not the type one would imagine would be interested in such literature'. He came to it, he told the officers, in search of enlightenment, and because 'his curiosity [was] aroused in childhood by not having sexual matters explained fully to him'.[16]

Others customers of Park Trading pleaded guilty to an equal amount of curiosity, while some claimed to have developed a sudden interest in photography or art. Inevitably, they were guarded when interviewed by the police, but their purchases say much about them. One man the police spoke to, a Cardiff steelworker whose address Park Trading had bought from another dealer, was fairly typical. His shopping list included not only a series of French and American pulps featuring naked women (not to mention ads for book dealers and lonely hearts clubs) such as *Amour de Paris*, *Free For All*, *Piccadilly Eyeful* and several others, but also 'anthropology' such as *Far Eastern Sex Life*, instruction in sex technique in the form of *Life Long Sex Harmony*, *Sex Instructions* and *Life Long Love*, and finally *The Truth About Nudism*.[17]

In fact, police inquiries into the obscenity trade showed again and again that the customers of porn dealers were not depraved or criminal as all the critics of obscene literature assumed, neither were they about to be corrupted. Instead they were generally very ordinary middle-class men, acting, they said, out of curiosity. We have to remember that for most of the twentieth century, official sex education scarcely existed either at home or at school. It was not until 1945 that sex education was recognised as a necessary component of the school curriculum, and even then it was left to the governors to decide whether they wanted it taught at their school. When it was taught, it could end up being couched in the form of awkward lectures on plant and animal biology. In this restricted climate, people who wanted to find explicit sources of information often had to look beyond school, family and friends and call on the help of the secretive networks of pornographers and book dealers. Once involved in this world, they became self-reliant and eclectic readers, treating sex as a field of knowledge to be carefully cultivated.

The Law of Hygiene for Our Wives, Being a New Treatise of Advice and information to married and those about to marry – send at once, medical catalogue enclosed.
My Pocket Novels, 1074, 1922

Before the 1960s, being a mail-order consumer in this way took a degree of effort. You had to educate yourself in the ways and codes of the market, seek out the best, least fraudulent dealers, establish a relationship of trust with them, and hope that their customer list was not confiscated by the police. When your books did arrive, you might find that what you thought was a racy work on fetishism or the female body turned out to be a history of flagellation or a treatise on the benefits of sunbathing. You might possibly be disappointed at first, but reading it – even for the wrong reasons – might mean that you learned something.

Chapter Seven

How Matrimonial Advertising (Nearly) Saved the Great British Marriage

In the spring of 1939, two former debutantes, Mary Oliver and Heather Jenner, were travelling back to Britain from Ceylon. Both came from wealthy, though not aristocratic families, some of whom were working for the Empire. Both were glamorous, pretty and twenty-five. They already knew each other slightly, but now, together on a ship for several weeks, they became friends and began to hatch a plan that they hoped would completely remake the marriage business and their own leisured lives.

Mary Oliver's own experiences in British India had partly prompted this decision. As a young, single woman visiting the colonies, she had inevitably been introduced to the most eligible bachelors in the district and had quickly become engaged to an older man. She had soon realised, however, that they were not suited to one another: he was on the look-out for a dutiful wife, while she was a resourceful and independent modern young woman. Tiring of his endless lectures on the responsibilities of marriage, she had ditched him and his expensive wedding plans and had taken a steamer for home. Now, returning to England, she realised that many of her fellow passengers gazing wistfully over the rails were single men, thinned by exile and starved of romance, who were going back to Britain after a period of colonial service in order to find a wife.

They would almost certainly get it wrong, she mused, proposing in haste to the first vaguely presentable girl they met and then repenting at leisure. It was a shame, she thought, that there was no better way of bringing these lonely colonials into contact with suitable girls who wanted a husband. Then she had a brainwave. Why not set up a business, a fashionable, refined matrimonial bureau, catering mainly for the upper classes, that would carefully and sensitively introduce potential partners to one another? Jenner, who later became the most famous marriage broker in Britain, thought at first that the whole thing was a joke, but soon Oliver's persistence and enthusiasm won her over.

In fact, Mary Oliver did have some prior experience of the matrimonial industry, but as a customer, not a proprietor. A few years before meeting Jenner, she had tried out the matrimonial press herself, partly to see if it worked. She had advertised for a husband, and soon found herself besieged by a steady stream of lower-middle-class suitors – bus drivers, commercial travellers, city clerks, sanitary inspectors and railwaymen. Much to her embarrassment, and the annoyance of her parents, these correspondents telephoned continually and even called at the house in person. The conclusion to be drawn was that there was clearly a market there, but that it did not cater for the wealthy and fashionable. What was required was a well-run organisation that could accommodate the upper classes – a more efficient version of the debutantes' 'season'. That, Mary Oliver judged, was not only a key part of the social calendar, but was not that different from a marriage market itself, since it involved 'parents spending fortunes to display their daughters impressively before supposedly eligible young men'.[1] An agency seemed to be the answer. Clients could be seen in person and given sympathetic, detailed and personal treatment. The agency would evalute them and then decide who on their books might make a suitable match. Interests, religious persuasion and, perhaps most importantly, social status and income would all be taken into consideration so that each marriage would start with 'a firm basis of equality and common interest'.[2]

For an enterprise such as this it was important to have a classy address, and so with a carefully hoarded capital of £50, Oliver and Jenner rented a Bond Street attic. At first it was furnished tastefully in soothing pastels to look like an upper-class drawing room, but both women soon realised that plain office decor was much more appropriate, as it suggested an atmosphere of businesslike objectivity. The Marriage Bureau was ready for business.

Charming spinster, really so, age 32, height 5 ft 3½ in, dark hair, blue eyes, bright complexion, beautiful voice and splendid pianoforte player, good income from own Studio, Church of England; wishes to meet Bachelor, 32 to 40, with income £600 or over.

Matchmaker, January 1928

Before long, their first customer arrived: a snobbish Indian Army officer looking for the sort of society wedding that would feature in *Tatler*, and that would allow him and his wife to return to India in triumph. Two months later, he was married. Within a month of its establishment the business was receiving 300 letters a day and troops of girls were making their way up the stairs of the Bond Street office, often nervous at first but soon given confidence by the calm, businesslike manner of the Bureau's two directors. As Jenner later recalled, the fact that they were also young, fashionable, 'frightfully nice' and did not look like crooks helped a great deal.

The Marriage Bureau may have been an instant commercial success but most of Jenner and Oliver's friends were horrified by it. They had imbibed the prejudices of the period, and assumed that the world of matrimonial agencies and small ads was one of fortune hunting, fraud and even white slavery. It certainly wasn't respectable, and it very definitely was not something done by nice upper-class girls. Jenner later recalled that when she started the business, most of her friends couldn't even bring themselves to speak about what she was doing. One of them ventured that because the two women were very young the excuse could be made for them that they were 'more mad than criminal' and added that they would almost certainly end up in trouble with the police. Attitudes changed though, 'when they found that we had not been carted off to prison for immoral behaviour and, on the contrary, were building up a good reputation'.[3]

By making the Marriage Bureau a fashionable upper-class concern, Jenner and Oliver virtually revolutionised the image of the matrimonial agency. Although several existed in the 1930s, and all of them had pretensions to the utmost respectability, they were rarely very discriminating about their clientele and so tended to have a poor reputation. The Marriage Bureau, by contrast, was socially exclusive. Advertising was placed not in newspapers or specialist journals set apart from the mainstream press, but in high-class magazines and theatre programmes. It also charged relatively high prices and used personal interviews to screen out undesirables.

The initial fee was 5 guineas, with a further 20 guineas to pay after a couple was married – quite a lot of money in 1939, when the average weekly income of a skilled worker was only £2 11s 6d. Not surprisingly, the fee structure ensured that only 15 per cent of the Bureau's customers could be described as working-class. The average income of clients was a very middle-class £500 per year. Most of them – more than 60 per cent – were between twenty-five and forty years old.[4]

Other factors contributed to the success of the Bureau. Since Jenner and Oliver received 80 per cent of the potential total fee only when a couple were actually married, it was in their interest to ensure that the relationships they promoted were likely to work. Fortune hunting was strictly discouraged, while those merely seeking sexual adventure were invariably deterred by the high prices and the laborious process of interview and questionnaire.

> Bachelor (Coloured), age 27, medium in height and build, good private income, living in London, educated and refined. Protestant: wishes to marry spinster, near own age, educated and broad-minded essential.
>
> *Matchmaker*, January 1928

Exclusive also meant white. The rare black visitor who had the courage to come to the Bureau in its early days was, Oliver recalled, shoved unceremoniously into a side room so that other clients would not think that he or she was representative of the potential brides or husbands on offer.[5] Jenner and Oliver were also adept at self-promotion, and instead of hiding away in shame at the unromantic nature of the enterprise, they actually courted press attention. Within a month of opening, the Bureau had been favourably puffed three times in the *Daily Mail* and written up by Godfrey Winn in the *Sunday Express*.[6]

Early success was boosted by the Second World War, even though the office had to be relocated away from London during the Blitz. By 1953, the Marriage Bureau was a well-established feature of upper-class society, had a branch in France, and claimed to have arranged over 5,000 marriages, only three of which had ended in divorce. Jenner reckoned that she had arranged at least one marriage a day for fourteen years. Clients included gentlemen of leisure, numerous middle-class professionals, opera singers, footballers, actresses and explorers – and four Members of Parliament. Jenner, whose publicity-seeking memoirs airbrushed out Oliver's early contribution (she left the business in 1942) with all the thoroughness of a Stalin, became a celebrity, making regular appearances at Butlin's holiday camp, as well as starring in the radio show *In Town Tonight* and the television panel game *What's My Line?*

Inventing the Matrimonial Agency

It had been a long road to respectability for the marriage business. Back in the 1690s, when it was first mentioned in the British press, it had been attacked as mercenary, fraudulent and, quite simply, unnecessary.[7] It had, however, survived initial hostility to become, by the early eighteenth century, a familiar feature of the new periodical press. Some of the early ads suggested something more than mere marriage, and instead offered ambiguous 'arrangements' in return for cash, perhaps as a cover for courtesans seeking clients. A few men clearly seemed to be advertising openly for mistresses or something similar, such as the 'Gentleman of independent fortune, in possession, and very considerable expectations' who intended to make a tour through France and Italy, with 'an agreeable young lady, whose education and sentiments would engage his esteem and affections'. Other men advertised for single women to board with them possibly as a way of making an informal marriage. Financial arrangements very much like prostitution were sometimes offered by women advertisers as well. One 1769 ad, to 'any real *gentleman*, from a *lady* of character', promised that in exchange for £100, a man could have 'an advantage, which cannot be named in a public newspaper'. Another who was 'at present so critically circumstanced as to want the immediate friendship and assistance of a gentleman of honour and benevolence', offered in return to 'render essential services'.[8]

In spite of these unconventional suggestions, most of the early ads were clearly matrimonial in intention, helping those without the necessary family connections to make a good marriage. Organised matrimonial agencies, such as the grandly titled Imprejudicate Nuptial Society, or the Grand Matrimonial Intercourse Institution, were also common in the eighteenth century.[9] However, in spite of the popularity of advertising, the usual requirement that advertisers declare their financial status in some detail gave the whole business a rather mercenary, unromantic feel. Nor was it helped by fears about the safety and status of single women, anxieties more than confirmed by the revelation that one of the most famous murderers of the nineteenth century, William Corder, who did away with his sweetheart Maria Marten at the infamous Red Barn at Polstead in Suffolk in 1828, had turned out to be a regular user of matrimonial ads.[10]

In spite of periodic scandals, and the continuing suspicion that the matrimonial press concealed fortune hunters, the industry nevertheless thrived in Victorian Britain. By 1900 there were twenty-five newspapers devoted to helping people find partners, and even though the marriage business was a regular subject for musical comedy, it had begun to attract a few powerful adherents. In 1897 a debate had begun in the fashionable women's magazine *The Woman at Home* over whether marriage would be helped by organised matrimonial bureaux, and the favourable response had encouraged W. T. Stead to start his matrimonial/social network the Wedding Ring Circle the following year. Even the ultra-respectable founder of the Salvation Army, William Booth, proposed that matrimonial bureaux might be employed to help the urban poor by taking them away from the the dangerous promiscuity of the streets and helping them to make suitable and healthy partnerships.[11]

By the inter-war period, some people were arguing that matrimonial agencies might be able to help with pressing demographic and cultural threats to the institution of marriage. Towards the end of the nineteenth century, birth rates had begun to fall, leading to anxiety over the potential decline in Britain's population and national strength. The idea of marriage was also changing – the Victorian notion that women should be essentially subordinate in marriage had begun to seem old-fashioned as far back as the 1880s, and by the 1920s seemed positively prehistoric. At the same time, a new atmosphere of sexual freedom, coupled with a post-war shortage of men and an economic depression that made it difficult for people to set up an independent home, meant that marriage was being left ever later. Observing the obstacles in the way of matrimony, and the evident scepticism with which the post-war generation treated the prospect of marriage, the radical American writer V. F. Calverton even went so far as to claim in 1929 that marriage was simply 'bankrupt'.[12] In 1851 men waited on average until they were twenty-five before they got married. By 1930 that figure had risen to twenty-seven. In the same period the average age at which women married rose from twenty-four to twenty-five.[13] The growing army of single people, combined with a widespread perception that traditional marriage was in some way inadequate, not only produced the lonely hearts industry but also stimulated a concerted debate about what form modern marriage should take.

Spinster at home every afternoon, age 30, fair complexion, medium height, good appearance, fond of sports and theatres, would meet gentleman of leisure, view matrimony.

The Times, 22 May 1928

The key question of the 1920s and 30s was how to reconcile the need to boost the birth rate with both traditional marriage and a growing belief among doctors and social reformers that a healthy sex life was fundamental to individual well-being. If most people were marrying in their mid- to late-twenties, that meant either people were having sex before marriage, which was generally regarded as either immoral or unhealthy, or they were staying celibate, which meant that they were being forced to deny a key aspect of their humanity. Some radicals dealt with the paradox by arguing against marriage altogether. The socialist philosopher Bertrand Russell and his wife Dora, for example, maintained that conventional marriage was an unnatural barrier to healthy sex. Others made the case for recognising and formalising extra-marital sex. Free love was put on the agenda (not for the first time), in the form of a 'contract partnership' model.[14] In this scheme, first proposed by the eugenicist Catherine Gasquoine Hartley in 1913, the state would intervene to allow unmarried men and women to set up households and have children by providing some kind of insurance in the event of a break-up. This arrangement would protect women from the insecurities of unregulated 'free love', while at the same time allowing those not suited to the constricting institution of marriage both to express their sexuality and to have children, thereby ensuring the future of the British race.[15] Contract partnerships, in Hartley's view, solved all the modern problems of sex and population by removing the insecurity of singleness and the stigma of illegitimacy while also protecting the birth rate. The overall aim of the scheme, like many other attempts to solve the problem of marriage in the 1920s and 30s, was to try and ensure the health of the race by maintaining the fertility of the 'racially fit' and enabling women to fulfil what Hartley felt was their reproductive destiny.[16] Others believed that marriage need not be rejected altogether but should be completely overhauled. One solution that was proposed by a few commentators in the 1920s and that was similar to Gasquoine Hartley's was to let people live with their partners in what was known as a 'trial marriage'. That idea, however, was dismissed by most as overly radical.[17] Yet another proposal, popular in progressive circles, was to develop a more 'companionate' model of legal marriage in which husband and wife entered into partnership as true equals and not with the man as the senior partner. Some, including the Russells, pushed the companionate model even further, arguing that a truly free marriage should also incorporate such modern ideas as birth control, divorce by mutual consent, and alimony in the event of separation.[18]

Against this background of debate and controversy, a consensus emerged about the need to prepare men and women for marriage through a process of 'marriage education', an idea that dated back to General Booth's welfare scheme of the 1890s. One advocate of companionate marriage argued in 1934 that in order to safeguard the health of the population and the future of the British race, the state should 'undertake the education of youth and married couples in the art of love, [and] the laws of sex life', in order to 'better equip them for the serious duties of marriage and parenthood'.[19] Marriage, it was maintained, could and should be taught in schools. By the 1930s, a loose coalition of leftist intellectuals, former social purity activists, eugenic theorists and Christian groups had come together in order to try and work out a programme of marriage education on these lines. Their solution to the 'problem' of marriage was a series of local organisations, set up throughout the country, which would help people through the difficulties of courtship and assist them as best they could to make healthy and successful marriages. This was the beginning of the movement for marriage guidance, and eventually, in 1946, it turned into the National Marriage Guidance Council (NMGC), now known as Relate.[20]

The Post-war Marriage Crisis

Britain in the years immediately after the Second World War was not a good time or place to be married. The divorce rate spiralled as large numbers of men and women returned from years of wartime separation to partners they hardly knew. Whereas there had been only 7,995 divorces in England and Wales in 1939, in 1947 there were over 60,000, a figure not matched again until 1971. The yearly average of petitions for divorce increased over five times from the pre-war figure to more than 38,000 between 1946 and 1950.[21] It is scarcely surprising therefore that fears should have been expressed for the future of marriage itself, or that the new Labour government should have turned to publicly funded marriage guidance as one solution to the crisis. Nor is it surprising, given the dislocation marriage had suffered, that matrimonial agencies like Heather Jenner's should have flourished anew, or that friendship clubs should have received a new lease of life. Some of this revival was centred on the kind of small-time operations which had been in business before the war, which now resumed with friendly names like the Two-Ways Contact Club, the Golden Circle Club, the Victory Correspondence Club, the Good Fellowship Club, the Friendship Circle, and the Friendly Folk Association, all of which emerged to cater for the single, the widowed or the lonely.

The classified ad also returned to prominence as one among

many possible solutions to the problem of meeting suitable partners. It still retained a somewhat tarnished image though, not helped by cases such as that of the 'lonely hearts killers' Raymond Fernandez and Martha Beck, who in 1948 defrauded and murdered a series of correspondence club members in the USA.[22] In spite of these horror stories, mainstream magazines got back into the market, not least the cinema fan magazine *Picture Show*, which ran a 'Star Fan Club' column that offered straight and gay readers a means of making contact with potential partners, even though male homosexuality remained a criminal offence. Sly references to one's love of the stars Farley Granger, Montgomery Clift or Bette Davis were apparently enough to signal a homoerotic intent, and sometimes to once again alert the police, especially when servicemen were involved.[23] Clubs and matrimonial agencies also sprang up across Europe, including one in Munich which was reported to have replaced photographs of its members with short films detailing their attributes. Even the BBC took notice, placing an ad in an evening paper for young women to meet a 'well-set up young man' outside the Criterion theatre, where, the following week, hundreds appeared to meet the advertiser. There were mixed reactions when the whole thing turned out to be a publicity stunt and it was realised that the young man in question was Brian Johnston, the presenter of the radio show *In Town Tonight.* The ensuing melee, in which Johnston was pursued across Piccadilly Circus by a

Friendly Folk Association. Social Introductions everywhere. Details free.

Writer, May 1949

crowd of both enthusiastic and mildly annoyed women, was broadcast live to the nation.[24]

Inevitably, the revival of 'friendship clubs' and companionship ads brought with it a fresh round of debate and criticism. The sociological survey Mass Observation looked at the friendship club boom, and concluded that, for the most part, operations like the Victory Correspondence Club did deliver what they promised.[25] At the other end of the scale, two novels of the period – Alan Wykes's *The Pen Friend* (1950) and Angus Wilson's *Hemlock and After* (1952) – both launched swingeing attacks on the companionship business, portraying advertisers as dupes, and proprietors as perverts or pornographers.[26] A more considered evaluation came in the spring of 1948, when, following a three-week investigation, the star tabloid reporter of the day, Douglas Warth, published a detailed report on post-war loneliness and the crisis of marriage in the *Sunday Pictorial*. To his surprise, he discovered that matrimonial agencies were more important than ever before, that they arranged an average of fifty-four marriages a month in London alone, and that Heather Jenner's Marriage Bureau had more than 2,000 marriages to its name. He was aware that agencies like this were open to abuse, and he felt that he couldn't recommend the industry as it was currently arranged, but he also recognised that it met the real needs of a large and hidden population of lonely people who desperately needed help.[27] Warth's recommendation was that society should tackle the huge problem of post-war loneliness by 'turning the whole business of arranged marriages into a social service'.[28]

Warth was not the only one to think that this was a matter of national importance. The first leader of the National

Marriage Guidance Council, an earnest and energetic former Methodist minister called David Mace, took a similar view. 'I don't need to tell you', Mace said in his 1948 book *Marriage Crisis*, 'that queer things are happening to marriage.' Not only was divorce more common ('Probably some of your friends are in the queue for the divorce court ... Perhaps yourself'), but, Mace argued, family breakdown was also a leading cause of juvenile crime.[29] Mace felt that anything which might help safeguard the future of marriage should be encouraged, even matrimonial agencies. He therefore set out to investigate the many matrimonial bureaux which already existed, to see whether they could form part of a much wider movement to save marriage and the nation's morals. In doing so, his efforts raised the matrimonial agency to new heights of respectability, and the combined arguments of Warth and Mace helped put the idea of state marriage agencies firmly onto the agenda.

Ex-Service woman, thirty-three, height 5ft. 5 in., fair, slim figure, rather reserved, wishes to meet bachelor thirty-five to forty, living in the Midlands.

Quoted in *Sunday Pictorial*, 28 March 1948

Mace's investigation – headlined a 'Specialist's Report' – appeared on 20 March 1948, at the height of the post-war marriage crisis. In a deliberate attempt to start a popular debate, the piece appeared as part of a series not in an academic journal but in the popular weekly *John Bull*.[30] Mace began by noting that although 'highly romantic' people might regard the idea of marriage agencies as distasteful, it was nevertheless time to give another, more scientific method a try. In the past ten years, he had received thousands of letters

A specialist's report on agencies that help people in the

SEARCH FOR A LIFE PARTNER

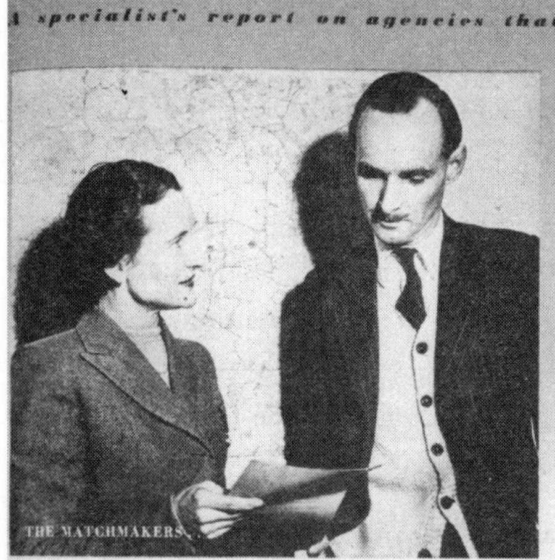

Lt.-Col. and Mrs. R. A. Cresswell, marriage bureau chiefs. Aim is to provide a needed social service

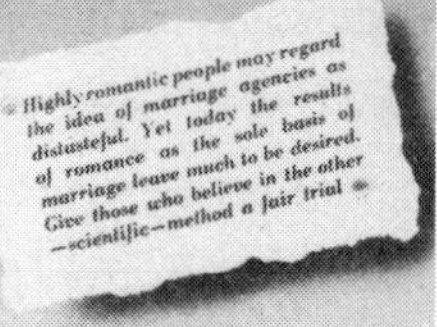

Highly romantic people may regard the idea of marriage agencies as distasteful. Yet today the results of romance as the sole basis of marriage leave much to be desired. Give those who believe in the other—scientific—method a fair trial

by Dr. DAVID MACE

Secretary, Marriage Guidance Council

IN THE PAST TEN YEARS I have received a great many letters from people who have asked me to help them find a suitable marriage partner. I should imagine they must run into many hundreds—possibly thousands.

These people have written without any encouragement from me; for I have never held out any prospect of being able to deal with this problem. They have written in desperation, as drowning men clutch at a straw.

Their need has haunted me. And the attitude of society to this problem has distressed me. When I have brought up the subject in discussion, most people have treated it as a joke. When I have assured them that I take an entirely serious view of the matter, they have suggested that I was being fooled by cranks who were imposing upon my goodwill.

I decided to put this accusation to the test. I picked on some of the people who had written to me, and investigated the facts about them. I made no selection—just chose one or two at random from the bunch. The result reassured me. They were shy people and lonely people; but they were certainly not cranks. Some of them were very fine people indeed.

Where's the Right Person?

There was a nice working man whose wife had been killed by a V2, leaving him with two small children. There was a professional man, a widower with a four-figure income, who was acutely lonely but had failed to find a woman whom he could ask to share his home. There was a cultured girl in the Civil Service who worked in an office full of women and seemed only to meet men of a type which she could not respect.

And there was a woman doctor whose men colleagues were all married already and who worked in a little town where the few eligible men would never have considered her as a possible wife.

All these people desperately wanted to marry. They were all in my opinion capable of becoming excellent husbands and wives. Yet their circumstances provided them with little opportunity to meet possible partners. And they could not easily change their circumstances.

Gradually I have come to see that human stories

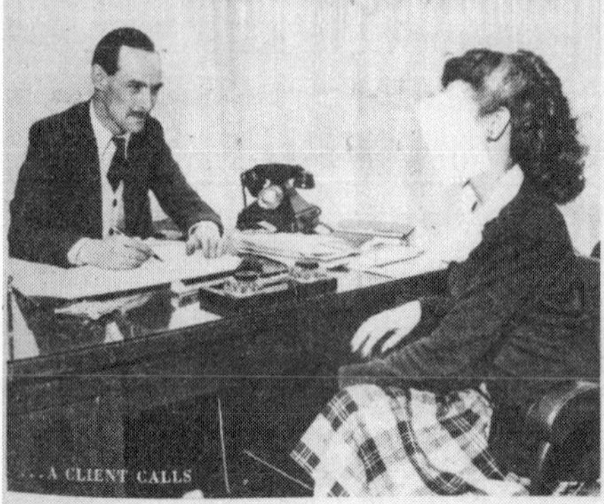

Interviews are confidential. Woman client gave special permission for this John Bull photograph

An article by David Mace, the first secretary of the Marriage Guidance Council, making the case for matrimonial bureaux and featuring Lt. Col. and Mrs R. A. Cresswell, proprietors of Marjorie Moore's marriage bureau (top right and left).

from lonely people looking for advice from an expert on how to find a life partner. A little investigation had shown him that these people – the natural market for the matrimonial agent and friendship club – were not cranks or failures, but ordinary, lonely people looking for a wife or husband. For Mace's correspondents it was almost impossible to meet people and build genuinely lasting ties of intimacy in the anonymous modern city. You could try going to dances, clubs or holiday camps, Mace said, but if you did, any relationships you formed would be on the basis only of an immediate and superficial attraction that might well prove an inadequate foundation for something lasting. There was a clear need, he argued, for a more formal and organised marriage bureau system, perhaps licensed or even established by the state.

Mace's conclusions were controversial. Instead of reporting the usual horror at the arrangement of marriages by third parties, a staple of press reporting since the eighteenth century, the sober Mace suggested that the matrimonial advertisement might, with state assistance, become a valuable social service and a suitable complement to the work of the NMGC. He singled out three agencies for particular praise: Heather Jenner and Mary Oliver's Marriage Bureau; Marjorie Moore's Marriage Bureau, which was a cheaper copy of Jenner's high-class operation, and was run from the Strand by an ex-Army officer; and the Bournemouth Marriage and Social Introduction Bureau, also run by a former military man. Another agency, the high-class Marriage Society, mimicked the NMGC even more closely, Mace said, since it employed highly qualified professionals and relied on extensive psychological profiling and scientific research in its attempts to match up ideal partners. There might be some agencies that operated purely for commercial gain but most of them were sound and should be welcomed. Instead of condemning people who met partners in this way, Mace argued that we should 'suspend judgment, and remember that in these days anything is to be welcomed which is likely to add to the total number of happy, stable marriages'. In another piece for *John Bull* the following May, Mace and his allies again urged that the NMGC should encourage the matrimonial bureaux to develop as a branch of social service and 'put their work on the highest possible level'.[31] There was a favourable public response to Mace's articles, especially from *John Bull*'s readers, many of whom demanded that the state set up its own network of matrimonial bureaux as part of the expanding apparatus of social care. 'We have welfare centres, mothercraft clinics, citizen's advice bureaux', one correspondent noted, so 'Why not a "Home-maker's office" in every town?'[32] The better class of agency also welcomed these suggestions, notably Lt. Col. R. A. Cresswell, proprietor of the Marjorie Moore agency, who told the *Sunday Pictorial* that in his view, 'marriage making should be State controlled'.[33] It seemed as though the long-despised matrimonial advertisement was about to receive its due, and might even become a key part of national policy.

The government, though, thought otherwise. It was not going to give money to an organisation, the NMGC, which seemed to have endorsed the morally dubious matrimonial ad as a solution to a national crisis. The whole thing, the government suggested, seemed to have originated in an unfortunate mixture of opportunism and lack of cash. Mace, one Home Office official concluded, had become 'too much addicted to publishing articles advertising himself and the NMGC with a view to getting money for the Council, whose finances have been, from the outset, in a very precarious state'.[34] Neither did the new Labour government want to associate its revolutionary welfare state with fly-by-night friendship clubs. After a brief investigation, the Home Office concluded that there was 'no conclusive evidence' that matrimonial bureaux were serving a socially useful purpose.[35] For that reason it was not possible to give government money to the NMGC unless it kept well away from marriage agencies.

Mace's colleagues also came out against his plan, arguing in time-honoured fashion that courtship by advertisement was only for those who had failed in life. Now, though, the rejection of the lonely heart had a gloss of psychological science. Mace's opponents didn't describe lonely advertisers merely as dupes, as had once been the case, nor did they argue that they were necessarily in moral danger, but the NMGC's final report did conclude that they were 'very susceptible to persuasion'. It argued that to let someone else choose a partner for you was 'a belittlement of personal responsibility', and that, in any case, people who relied on external expertise to find a partner probably lacked the necessary flexibility and character required for a successful marriage. The ups and downs of ordinary courtship, it was argued, naturally prepared potential spouses for the give and take of marriage, and that could not be artificially replicated by a marriage broker.[36]

Internal politics played a part in the rejection of Mace's scheme. The NMGC was concerned to defend its own expertise in the area of marriage guidance, and to deter commercial operations from copying its methods. It was also acutely aware that government funding was at stake, and that it faced competition from many other organisations seeking state funding. It had, therefore, to make every effort to distinguish itself from its cousins in the matrimonial industry. Consequently Mace's attempt to make common cause with the matrimonial agency eventually came to nothing.

For a brief moment, though, the once-despised business of matrimonial advertising had seemed to offer a popular, user-friendly and, above all, respectable solution to the post-war problem of marriage. The solid Colonel Cresswell, of the Majorie Moore agency, and the highbrow Marriage Society of Harley Street appeared, even to serious social reformers like David Mace, to offer a true social service, a potentially more popular answer to contemporary problems than the paternalistic NMGC and its eugenist-religious allies.

> Are you lonely? I know just the person who would make you happy. Somewhere your ideal husband or wife is waiting – still a complete stranger. Let me introduce you. Write giving particulars of yourself and the sort of person you would like to marry. Send stamped addressed envelope for full details.
>
> Quoted in *Sunday Pictorial*, 28 March 1948

After 1947, however, marriage guidance and the matrimonial industry diverged, never to meet again. While Jenner's business continued to prosper right up to the 1970s, and she remained a minor celebrity, the Marriage Bureau and its ilk never again assumed a position at the cutting edge of contemporary debate. As for the NMGC, it soon shifted its emphasis from training *for* marriage to settling disputes *between* those already married. It also distanced itself from its origins as a grass-roots movement of willing amateurs and increasingly required all counsellors to have academic training in psychology.

In any case, by the mid-1950s, the marriage crisis was over. Full employment, affluence, and the end of the wartime housing shortage meant that it became easier to establish a separate household away from one's parents, and as a result, more people than ever were getting married. The big church wedding was back, and marriage became practically compulsory for the young.[37] The average age of marriage fell accordingly. By 1958 it had fallen to 25 for men, its lowest since 1880, and to 22.6 for women, the lowest since the census of 1851.[38] The services of the marriage broker and the introduction agency no longer seemed so necessary, and they were now to be found most conspicuously in the new immigrant communities from India and Pakistan. It was, however, the sexual revolution of the next decade that was really to send matrimonial advertising back to the edge of cultural debate.

Chapter Eight

Contact: Wife Swapping and the Contradictions of Sexual Revolution

Edward Donelly was a small-time crook, and although he was only twenty-four, he had managed to run up a fairly substantial criminal record. Now, though, he was going straight – in a way. He and an associate, James Mcguigan, had gone into journalism, buying two small, cheap, but promising magazines from a mate and running them from a dingy lock-up in a West London mews. This was Notting Hill in the 1960s, a place very far from the funkily gentrified streets depicted in the 1999 film that still draws tourists from around the world to the chi-chi shops and cafes of the Portobello Road. While Donelly's lock-up is probably now one of the more expensive pieces of real estate in London, in the 1950s and 60s this part of West London was a tough neighbourhood whose huge stuccoed villas were divided into ever-smaller bedsits and shabby flats by unscrupulous rack-renting slumlords. Many of these were let to the West Indian immigrants who had come to the area in the 1950s, and who had been the target of race riots in 1958. In contrast, some houses were pop-star bolt-holes, like the Hotel Samarkand in Ladbroke Grove where Jimi Hendrix overdosed in 1969, while others were squatted by clans of aspiring bohemians. Donelly and Mcguigan were part of this clashing world of hippies, racial tension and peeling paint, as indicative of the 1960s as any icon of flower power and swinging London.

Although theirs was an unglamorous and even seedy world, Donelly and Mcguigan were as much part of the sexual revolution of the 1960s as any advocate of free love, for both men were in the swinging business. They were the editors and printers of *Exit* and *Way Out*, two of many small and short-lived titles that emerged in the late 1960s to try and make some money by putting the supposedly freewheeling sexuality of the times into practice. The two magazines contained contact ads from those interested in exploring what in the late 1960s – sexual revolution notwithstanding – still constituted the outer reaches of sexual behaviour.

Both *Exit* and *Way Out* were small-format and poorly printed. They lured their readers with covers featuring naked women posing in outdoor settings and contained around 300 ads offering various kinds of sexual experimentation. In addition, a commercial section was devoted to the needs and wants of amateur pornographers, dealers in films and photographs, and home-made erotica obtainable via the Man U Script Club. Other ads, much like those that appeared in the columns of *London Life* in the 1920s, offered private collections of cuttings and photographs concerned with 'rubber, leather, costume, tight lacing, Riding kit uniforms, CP TV' and other 'unusual items'. A handful dealt with more practical matters, such as the one proclaiming the benefits of 'Magnaphall', an allegedly 'absolutely safe' and 'sound and successful method of increasing the size of the male organ and enhancing virility'.[1]

It was the classified contact ads, however, that were the main selling point for both *Exit* and *Way Out*. At £1 for a minimum of twenty-four words you could join the sexual revolution – a rate that, Donelly told his readers, was extremely competitive. After all, he said, why spend as much as £5 in some tawdry dive in the West End just for the privilege of having a girl sit with you while you sipped overpriced cider masquerading as champagne, when for the same amount you could send five letters to some new and exciting friends who might offer the prospect of a much more authentic encounter. These ads offered an outlet not only to the fantasies of cost-conscious heterosexual men, but also to those who felt marginalised by the main currents of sexual revolution – gay men (and some women), those into fetish or S&M, suburban married couples seeking adventure, transvestites and transgender people – indeed almost everyone who wanted to join in the sexual revolution but who could find no real home among a hippy counterculture which claimed to be radical and to welcome everyone, but in practice remained youthfully cliquey, male-dominated and aggressively heterosexual. Some gay ads were straightforward appeals for friendship and sex, such as that from 'Executive type male 51, single, fair, slim build, bright personality', who sought 'another for lasting friendship and mutual pleasure, (Berks)'. Others struck a rather more mercenary note, such as that from 'Youth 21, versatile slim attractive English', who offered 'full personal services to gentlemen of any age, at my place or yours'. Among the more esoteric was one promising 'pleasurable company occasional mornings or afternoons' to 'really overweight ladies', while another from 'Indian, 25, versed in Indian arts' offered

> Clean, good looking man, 44, prepared to satisfy any ladies wishes, completely safe. Monmouthshire and Birmingham.
> *Exit*, 38, 1968

seminars for 'older couples to add spice to life . . . No fees. (Scotland)'. Provincial swingers distanced from the world of metropolitan sophistication were represented by the 'Happily Married Couple 38/25, attractive', who 'would like to meet others for fun and friendship in North Devon'.[2]

In spite of the outlandish nature of some of the ads he carried, Donelly must have been pretty confident that his whole operation was legally above board. After all, male homosexuality between consenting adults in private had been legalised in 1967, so allowing advertising for same-sex partners should, theoretically, no longer have carried the same danger it once did. As a result, Donelly was surprised, one morning in October 1968, to receive a visit from the police. They had become aware of *Exit* and *Way Out* and had decided that both publications were obscene. Donelly protested loudly against what he clearly felt was harassment. At this time both magazines were selling about 9,000 copies a month and, according to the police, bringing in around £100 a day, so he had a lot of money riding on the enterprise. 'I shall fight this', he told the officer leading the raid, 'I've got a lot of money tied up in this business and I'll ask for it to be put before a jury.'[3] He said he knew that there had been a magazine called *Continental Way Out* that had got into trouble in the past, but that had nothing to do with him. He also said that he was careful to check all the ads he ran and take out any that he thought were 'dirty'. Like Alfred Barrett before him, Donelly thought that *Exit*, far from being an obscene publication, 'served a useful purpose'. Unfortunately, like Barrett, his view differed from that of the authorities, and Donelly and Mcguigan were duly charged with conspiring to corrupt public morals.

Ever since the *Link* case in 1921, the police had tended to clamp down on any publication which could be suspected of harbouring the ads of prostitutes or homosexuals. Their instrument was the vague and ancient common-law offence of conspiring to corrupt public morals, which, though rarely used in the twentieth century, was employed several times to attack publications that seemed to advertise prostitution. The *Ladies' Directory*, a compilation of ads for Soho prostitutes, had been prosecuted successfully in 1960, while gay contact ads had got the hippy paper *International Times* (*IT*) into trouble in 1966. Legal experts, including the defence in the *Ladies' Directory* case who took it all the way to the Court of Appeal, argued that the charge was archaic and did not actually describe any offence. However, in the case of *Exit* and *Way Out*, the Obscene Publications Squad knew that their actions had more than one precedent, and acted accordingly.[4] Their inquiries focused mainly on whether or not Donelly and Mcguigan were actually facilitating prostitution, and if the police could warn off gay advertisers, so much the better. The case, largely focusing on whether the charge actually existed, dragged its way through the courts, eventually reaching the House of Lords on appeal in the summer of 1972, at which point the two men were finally convicted. *Exit* and *Way Out*, and their advertisers, were judged to have corrupted the public.

Sex, Small Ads, and the Counterculture

Donelly and Mcguigan were, in spite of appearances, directly involved with the complicated sexual revolution of 1960s

Britain. By 1968, when the two men were arrested, their magazines could be taken as part of the general revolt against conventional morality among the young. By that time, the hippy underground, increasingly styling itself as the counter-culture, had created a powerful rhetoric of sexual freedom, one which preached the liberation of desire and the equality of passions, and recognised the need to start the revolution from within by liberating the mind from Victorian repressions. Everyone should be free to do anything, it was held, and they should be equally free to do it. As Emmanuel Petrakis, the co-founder of the UK-based Sexual Emancipation Movement put it in *IT* in 1969, Western society was only just emerging from 'the Dark Ages of Puritanism' which had held the Anglo-Saxon world in its icy grip. Unhappy love lives, he said, led to unconscious complexes and repressions, which in turn provoked wars, famines and social crisis. To counter this heritage of negativity, sexual revolutionaries should try to be naked wherever possible, and to cuddle people instead of saying hello. Men had to 'try not to be selfish' and to ensure that women gained pleasure, too. Another *IT* columnist proclaimed the benefits of 'MAGICAL LOVEMAKING', during which the conscious mind could 'integrate more deeply with our submerged consciousness' through the means of a 'super orgasm'.[5] Women's role in this brave new world was somewhat equivocal, however, and was summed up by the Petrakis manifesto. While men, it was assumed, could be trusted to embrace free love with gusto, women were enjoined to overcome their inhibitions and 'learn to give of yourselves a bit more (with adequate contraception)'. Even if they didn't enjoy it at first, Petrakis said, 'why not give pleasure to others?'[6]

In other words, although the public message from a Yippie pamphlet was that 'people should fuck all the time, whomever they wish', much of the sexual side of the counterculture was actually a celebration of phallic, male, heterosexuality.[7]

The response of many of those alienated by this aspect of the counterculture was, at the start of the 1970s, to set up their own political movements, most notably Women's Liberation and the Gay Liberation Front (GLF). Less political souls, however, were left to seek different outlets. And for some of them, the classified listings pioneered by underground papers like *Exit* and *IT*, and *Time Out* (then a poster-sized ad sheet) turned out to be more promising sources of personal freedom than the often overblown rhetoric of a hippy editorial or a sex guru's pamphlet. Ads and listings which appeared in the underground press were not only about sex, but also gave a sense of coherence to the counterculture and the gay scene of the 1970s. News sheets like *Time Out* and *Alternative London*, with their endless columns of classifieds and little ads promoting concerts, events, meetings, sit-ins and be-ins, provided the best guide to the counterculture because they did not just tell you about the underground, or philosophise about it, like *IT* and the hippy press, but actually showed you how to join the 'alternative' community.[8]

Just as they had since the Edwardian period, small ads continued to play a key role in the formation of the gay scene. Many gay men, in fact, preferred the neutral territory of the personal column to the overly political and confrontational message of Gay Liberation. Gay ads appeared regularly in *IT*, which had a special 'Gentlemen's Directory' section at the back to cater for them. *Exit* and *Way Out* also catered for

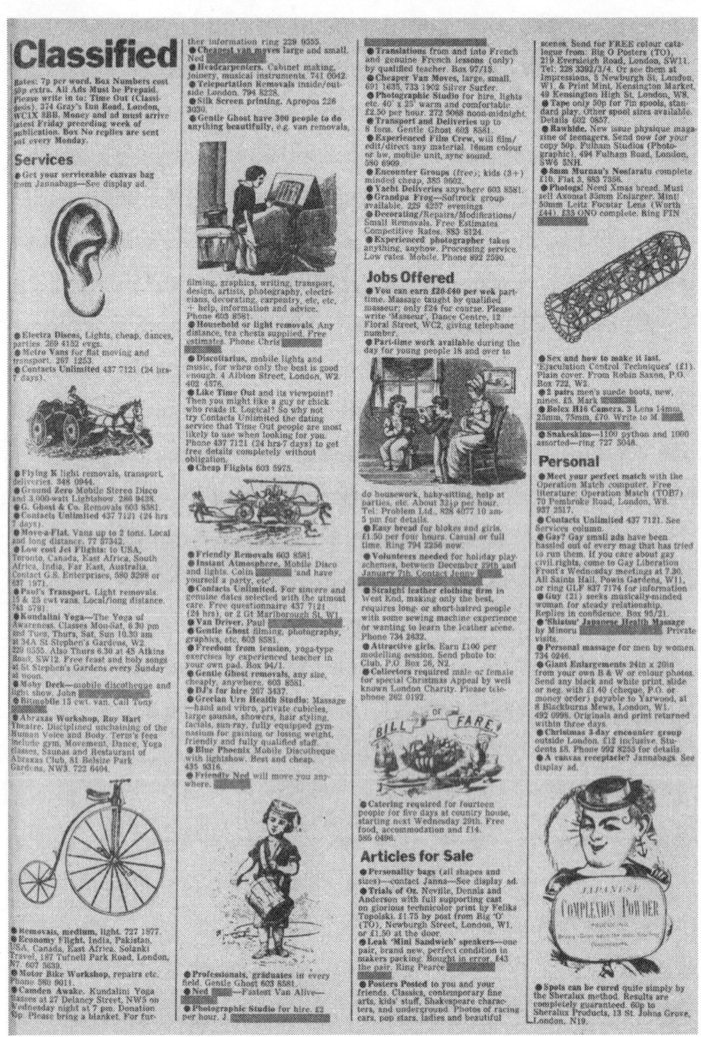

Classified

Rates: 7p per word. Box Numbers cost 10p extra. All Ads Must be Prepaid. Please write in to: Time Out (Classifieds), 374 Gray's Inn Road, London, WC1X 8BB. Money and ad must arrive latest Friday preceding week of publication. Box No replies are sent out every Monday.

Services

● Get your serviceable canvas bag from Jannabags—See display ad.

● **Electra Discos.** Lights, cheap, dances, parties. 269 4152 evgs.
● **Metro Vans** for flat moving and transport. 267 1253.
● **Contacts Unlimited** 437 7121 (24 hrs-7 days).

● **Flying K** light removals, transport, deliveries. 348 0944.
● **Ground Zero** Mobile Stereo Disco and 3,000-watt Lightshow. 286 9438.
● **G. Ghost & Co.** Removals 603 8581.
● **Contacts Unlimited** 437 7121 (24 hrs 7 days).
● **Move-a-Flat.** Vans up to 2 tons. Local and long distance. 77 57342.
● **Low cost Jet Flights:** to USA, Toronto, Canada, East Africa, South Africa, India, Far East, Australia. Contact G.S. Enterprises, 580 3298 or 637 1971.
● **Paul's Transport.** Light removals. 15 & 25 cwt vans. Local/long distance. 743 5781.
● **Kundalini Yoga**—The Yoga of Awareness. Classes Mon-Sat, 6.30 pm and Tues, Thurs, Sat, Sun 10.30 am at 34A St Stephen's Gardens, W2. 229 8555. Also Thurs 6.30 at 45 Atkins Road, SW12. Free feast and holy songs at St Stephen's Gardens every Sunday at noon.
● **Moby Deck**—mobile discotheque and light show. John
● **Bitmobile** 15 cwt. van. Call Tony

● **Abraxas Workshop, Roy Hart** Theatre. Disciplined unchaining of the Human Voice and Body. Term's fees include gym, Movement, Dance, Yoga classes, Saunas and Restaurant of Abraxas Club, 81 Belsize Park Gardens, NW3. 722 6404.

● **Removals, medium, light.** 727 1877.
● **Economy Flight.** India, Pakistan, USA, Canada, East Africa. Solanki Travel, 187 Tufnell Park Road, London, N7. 607 5639.
● **Motor Bike Workshop,** repairs etc. Phone 380 9011.
● **Camden Awake.** Kundalini Yoga classes at 27 Delancy Street, NW5 on Wednesday night at 7 pm. Donation 5p. Please bring a blanket. For further information ring 229 0555.
● **Cheapest van moves** large and small. Ned
● **Headcarpenters.** Cabinet making, joinery, musical instruments. 741 0042.
● **Teleportation Removals** inside/outside London. 794 8228.
● **Silk Screen printing.** Apropos 226 3030.
● **Gentle Ghost have 300 people to do anything beautifully,** e.g. van removals, filming, graphics, writing, transport, design, artists, photography, electricians, decorating, carpentry, etc. etc. + help, information and advice. Phone 603 8581.
● **Household or light removals.** Any distance, tea chests supplied. Free estimates. Phone Chris
● **Discotlarius,** mobile lights and music, for when only the best is good enough. 4 Albion Street, London, W2. 402 4378.
● **Like Time Out** and its viewpoint? Then you might like a guy or chick who reads it. Logical? So why not try Contacts Unlimited the dating service that Time Out people are most likely to use when looking for you. Phone 437 7121 (24 hrs-7 days) to get free details completely without obligation.
● **Cheap Flights** 603 5975.

● **Friendly Removals** 603 8581.
● **Instant Atmosphere.** Mobile Disco and lights. Colin 'and have yourself a party, etc'
● **Contacts Unlimited.** For sincere and genuine dates selected with the utmost care. Free questionnaire 437 7121 (24 hrs), or 2 Gt Marlborough St, W1.
● **Van Driver.** Paul
● **Gentle Ghost** filming, photography, graphics, etc. 603 8581.
● **Freedom from tension,** yoga-type exercises by experienced teacher in your own pad. Box 94/1.
● **Gentle Ghost removals,** any size, cheaply, anywhere. 603 8581.
● **DJ's for hire** 267 3437.
● **Grecian Urn Health Studio:** Massage—hand and vibro, private cubicles, large saunas, showers, hair styling, facials, sun-ray, fully equipped gymnasium for gaining or losing weight, friendly and fully qualified staff.
● **Blue Phoenix** Mobile Discotheque with lightshow. Best and cheap. 435 9316.
● **Friendly Ned** will move you anywhere.

● **Professionals, graduates** in every field. Gentle Ghost 603 8581.
● **Ned** —Fastest Van Alive—
● **Photographic Studio** for hire. £2 per hour. J.
● **Translations** from and into French and genuine French **lessons** (only) by qualified teacher. Box 97/13.
● **Cheaper Van Moves,** large, small. 691 1635, 733 1902 Silver Surfer.
● **Photographic Studio** for hire, lights etc. 40' x 25' warm and comfortable £2.50 per hour. 272 5068 noon-midnight.
● **Transport and Deliveries** up to 8 tons. Gentle Ghost 603 8581.
● **Experienced Film Crew,** will film/edit/direct any material. 16mm colour or b/w, mobile unit, sync sound. 580 6909.
● **Encounter Groups** (free); kids (3+) minded cheap. 385 0602.
● **Yacht Deliveries** anywhere 603 8581.
● **Grandpa Frog**—Softrock group available. 229 4257 evenings.
● **Decorating/Repairs/Modifications/** Small Removals. Free Estimates. Competitive Rates. 885 8124.
● **Experienced photographer** takes anything, anyhow. Processing service. Low rates. Mobile. Phone 892 2590.

Jobs Offered

● **You can earn £20-£40 per wek** part-time. Massage taught by qualified masseur; only £24 for course. Please write 'Masseur', Dance Centre, 12 Floral Street, WC2, giving telephone number.
● **Part-time work available** during the day for young people 18 and over to do housework, baby-sitting, help at parties, etc. About 32½p per hour. Tel: Problem Ltd., 828 4077 10 am-5 pm for details.
● **Easy bread** for blokes and girls. £1.50 per four hours. Casual or full time. Ring 794 2256 now.
● **Volunteers needed** for holiday playschemes, between December 29th and January 7th. Contact Jenny
● **Straight leather clothing firm** in West End, making only the best, requires long- or short-haired people with some sewing machine experience or wanting to learn the leather scene. Phone 734 2632.
● **Attractive girls.** Earn £100 per modelling session. Send photo to: Club, P.O. Box 26, N2.
● **Collectors** required male or female for special Christmas Appeal by well known London Charity. Please telephone 262 0192.

● **Catering** required for fourteen people for five days at country house, starting next Wednesday 29th. Free food, accommodation and £14. 586 0494.

Articles for Sale

● **Personality bags** (all shapes and sizes)—contact Janna—See display ad.
● **Trials of Oz.** Neville, Dennis and Anderson with full supporting cast on glorious technicolor print by Feliks Topolski. £1.75 by post from Big 'O' (TO), Newburgh Street, London, W1, or £1.50 at the door.
● **Leak 'Mini Sandwich' speakers**—one pair, brand new, perfect condition in makers packing. Bought in error, £43 the pair. Ring Pearce
● **Posters Posted** to you and your friends. Classics, contemporary fine arts, kids' stuff, Shakespeare characters, and underground. Photos of racing cars, pop stars, ladies and beautiful scenes. Send for FREE colour catalogue from: Big O Posters (TO), 219 Eversleigh Road, London, SW11. Tel: 228 3392/3/4. Or see them at Impressions, 5 Newburgh St, London, W1, & Print Mint, Kensington Market, 49 Kensington High St, London, W8.
● **Tape** only 50p for 7in spools, standard play. Other spool sizes available. Details 602 0857.
● **Rawhide.** New issue physique magazine of teenagers. Send now for your copy 50p. Fulham Studios (Photographic), 494 Fulham Road, London, SW6 5NH.
● **8mm Murnau's Nosfaratu** complete £10. Flat 3, 883 7356.
● **Photogs!** Need Xmas bread. Must sell Axomat 35mm Enlarger. Mint! 50mm Leitz Focotar Lens (Worth £44), £35 ONO complete. Ring FIN

● **Sex and how to make it last.** 'Ejaculation Control Techniques' (£1). Plain cover. From Robin Saxon, P.O. Box 722, W3.
● **2 pairs** men's suede boots, new, nines. £5. Mark
● **Bolex H16 Camera.** 3 Lens 14mm, 25mm, 75mm, £70. Write to M.
● **Snakeskins**—1100 python and 1000 assorted—ring 727 5048.

Personal

● **Meet your perfect match** with the Operation Match computer. Free literature: Operation Match (TOB7) 70 Pembroke Road, London, W8. 937 2517.
● **Contacts Unlimited** 437 7121. See Services column.
● **Gay?** Gay small ads have been hassled out of every mag that has tried to run them. If you care about gay civil rights, come to Gay Liberation Front's Wednesday meetings at 7.30, All Saints Hall, Powis Gardens, W11, or ring GLF 837 7174 for information.
● **Guy** (21) seeks musically-minded woman for steady relationship. Replies in confidence. Box 95/21.
● **'Shiatsu' Japanese Health Massage** by Minoru Private visits.
● **Personal massage** for men by women. 734 0246.
● **Giant Enlargements** 24in x 20in from your own B & W or colour photos. Send any black and white print, slide or neg. with £1.40 (cheque, P.O. or money order) payable to Yarwood, at 8 Blackburns Mews, London, W1. 492 0998. Originals and print returned within three days.
● **Christmas 3-day encounter group** outside London. £12 inclusive. Students £8. Phone 992 8255 for details.
● **A canvas receptacle?** Jannabags. See display ad.

● **Spots can be cured** quite simply by the Sheralux method. Results are completely guaranteed. 60p to Sheralux Products, 13 St. Johns Grove, London, N19.

A page of classified ads from the early days of Time Out – *December 1971.*

advertisers like the 'Continental fellow 22 years' looking for 'tall gay friends', and 'Sincere young gentleman' seeking 'male companionship, late twenties, perhaps flatshare'.[9] *Jeffrey*, one of the first wholly gay magazines in Britain, which was founded in 1972 as an alternative to the GLF periodical *Come Together*, promoted both 'Photo Pen Pals' and 'Jeffrey's Little Ads' for men like the Lancashire advertiser who was 'Gay But Not Screaming, well-built and interested in corresponding with male aged 21–26'. Soon, *Jeffrey* had its own 'Pen Partner Club' fulfilling the 'great need for gay people to communicate with each other' in order to find friends and lovers.[10]

Small ads didn't only cater for the newly visible gay scene, but also promoted other forms of sexual experimentation. To those who felt sexually adventurous but slightly at odds with the spirit of the times, such as the married, suburban, middle-aged, or politically conservative, small ads like those in *Exit* and *Way Out* could provide access to wife swapping, group sex and swinging. *Way Out* in particular catered for many of these homespun versions of the sexual revolution, advertising in 1967 the H Circle Club of genteel Muswell Hill, 'For Broad-minded Adult Males Only', and other clubs for the 'Broadminded Swinging Set'. Numerous other individual ads offered various forms of group sex or partner exchange, such as that promised by the 'Attractive educated couple 27/30', who expressed a 'desire to meet similar couples interested

> Torbay area. Sincere couple 38/28 interested in absolutely everything erotic wish to meet others similar for anything goes. Hurry we are so bored down here and very genuine.
>
> *Correspondent* 19, 1969

films, photos and fun activities . . .' or the 'Group being formed. Yorks/Teeside/Durham/Marrieds, singles', that requested 'details, preferences, photo etc. All types considered (Teeside)'.[11]

Even though these ads existed in quite large numbers, swinging and wife swapping have come to represent the failure of the sexual revolution of the 1960s. The British and American swinging scene of the early 1970s with its singles bars and bourgeois key parties seems like a poor rerun of the original sexual revolution of the 1960s, a dreadful alienated echo of the counterculture's high ideals.[12] Rick Moody's 1994 Nixon-era novel *The Ice Storm*, in which two sets of troubled parents attend a depressing swingers' party with their friends while their unsupervised children go off the rails, crystallised this image of the sixties' aftermath. However, perhaps swinging has been imperfectly remembered, and we should see suburban wife swapping and group sex in the same terms as the free love of the counterculture, something equally characteristic of the 1960s. After all, if the sexual revolution was going to succeed, then it would have to spread beyond the radical and mainly metropolitan vanguard who espoused it. So who were the wife swappers, and, more importantly, did they really exist?

The Origins of Wife Swapping

Wife swapping, or swinging, as its advocates preferred to call it, was another American import to sixties Britain, and like many of the phenomena borrowed by the British at the time, including the counterculture itself, it was perhaps done more thoroughly and extensively on the other side of the Atlantic. Most people probably still think of swinging as its early investigators did – as a kind of semi-mythical act, a rumoured pastime that probably never took place in the same liberated way as its supposed participants claimed. When the American anthropologist Gilbert Bartell set out to investigate the swinging scene in 1969, he posed the same questions which we might ask today: was it a myth, or did it actually take place? If so, who did it, and how many of them were there? Was it organised or merely the isolated practice of a few people? How did they meet? Were they actually lonely 'perverts' or hippy radicals? Inquiries like these alerted people in Britain to the fact that it might be happening here.

What first brought swinging to public notice in America was a sensational series run by the pin-up magazine *Mr* in 1957, purporting to show that it was a widespread practice and asking for accounts of readers' experiences. The magazine then ran a survey based on a reader questionnaire and published the results. Perhaps unsurprisingly, since *Mr* had a vested interest in both titillating its readers and encouraging them to be the sexual athletes they imagined themselves to be, the survey revealed that swinging was much more widespread than most people believed. *Wife Swapping*, the 1965 book compiled from the *Mr* survey and other sources, showed that swinging predated the 1960s, and had antecedents in the 'adultery toleration' pacts and open marriages that had been a feature of progressive sexual relations as far back as the 1920s. One reader even claimed that he had encountered a version of wife swapping in the American south-west at that time. Lonely air-force bases in 1950s Florida were also supposedly hotbeds of swinging and amateur pornography. By 1961, innocuous ads appearing in the *San Francisco Chronicle* from 'broad minded' couples new to the Bay Area were said to be coded invitations to 'sex orgies placed by the radical Sexual Freedom League'.[13]

Following the *Mr* survey, revelatory articles on the swinging scene became a regular feature of girlie mags and eventually made their way into the mainstream press. The first efforts to map the scene came from sensational paperbacks with titles like *The Velvet Underground* (1963), *The Sex Rebels* (1964) and *Mate-Swapping Syndrome* (1967), stories that were soon joined by serious-sounding books such as William and Jerrye Breedlove's *Swap Clubs: A Study in Contemporary Sexual Mores* (1964).[14] In 1967 the *Chicago Daily News* ran a series of articles condemning a local group of wife swappers as psychologically deviant, while almost simultaneously two separate groups of graduate students began to compile evidence on the subject. The first MA thesis on swinging was submitted at the University of California at Riverside in the same year. In 1970, the inaugural National Swingers' Convention, attended by 184 couples, was held in that alleged den of deviance, Chicago. By 1971, wife swapping had reached the pages of the *New York Times*, had been welcomed as a form of sexual liberation in Edward Brecher's history of sexology *The Sex Researchers* (1970), and had inspired the most complete investigation of the subculture, Gilbert Bartell's *Group Sex: A Scientist's Report on the American Way of Swinging.*[15]

All those writing about swinging agreed that it relied on contacts made through classified ads that appeared in a wide variety of magazines and newspapers. These ads had started appearing as far back as 1955 in an American paper called *La Plume*. While Brecher and others assumed that most of the early ads in papers like this were fakes, put in by the editors of girlie mags to try and prove to their readers that they weren't alone in their fantasies, they soon inspired more genuine attempts to bring swingers together. By the early 1960s there were around twenty magazines in America, Canada and Europe that published swingers' ads, and by 1970 there were more than thirty.[16] The 'Attractive couple in late 30s, she 5' 7", 145 [lbs], 38-23-38, he 6', 180 [lbs]' interested in 'conversation, cocktails and swinging interests', or the 'discreet couple' after similarly 'discreet, kind and broad-minded couples of any age for fun and pleasure' were typical of most serious advertisers. Vital statistics, especially of the female partner, were de rigueur.[17] Some of the magazines which carried these ads, like *Kindred Spirits* or *Swingers' Life*, were solely devoted to the scene, but ads also appeared in a slew of girlie mags and in supermarket tabloids like the *National Informer*. When the scene was still in its early days, one editor decided to advertise a party for swingers, which to his amazement was attended not by a gang of way-out sexual outlaws or single male perverts, but by more than 100 ordinary-looking heterosexual couples. Other papers followed suit, bringing their swinging readers into an embryonic community.[18]

In 1969, *Playboy* magazine reported from the heart of the Californian swinging scene that 'a new breed of unabashed orgiasts and casual couplers' was flourishing in its liberal climate. *Playboy*, whose guiding principle was to sell the sexual revolution not merely as personal liberation but also as a glamorous and seductive lifestyle, portrayed the high-class swinging scene as something which went naturally with wealth, status and the most refined kind of taste. At a glass and stucco house perched in the Hollywood Hills high above LA, the magazine reported, a retired businessman was preparing his annual New Year's orgy. In an open-plan room, a dozen unmarried couples passed round joints 'of the best available marijuana – Acapulco Gold – while they gazed at the incomparable view of the twinkling city lights visible through a picture window' and ate exotic middle-eastern delicacies prepared by the host. Before long, they were all thrashing around naked in a simulacrum of the *Playboy* mansion, a dimly lit bedroom which overlooked 'a lush garden of Japanese ferns, bonsais and camellias surrounding a heated pool stocked with exotic tropical fish'. Soon they were making love with an imagination and diversity that was as satisfying and 'as rich as the sumptuous buffet'. In another nearby house of a TV personality, jeroboams of Dom Perignon and twelve-year-old Scotch were poured by uniformed waiters, while the guests were put into the mood by the soothing strings of Mantovani. It was the kind of place where you might even meet a star of the moment, someone like Mia Farrow, who told *Playboy* that she had been taken to swinging parties by Salvador Dali but had only watched, sensing that the whole thing was an elaborate performance, not unlike a ballet.[19]

Playboy, with its fascination for interiors, architecture and all the paraphernalia of sophistication, provided a seductive image of the swinging scene. But was swinging really all about champagne and Mantovani? Or was it a rather tamer and less exotic affair, as more sober accounts suggested? It was in order to get at the truth of this that the anthropologist Gilbert Bartell and his (unnamed) wife set out to compile an exhaustive study in the late 1960s. The Bartells posed as a willing couple new to the scene and found a way in to the swinging networks of the Chicago area, answering ads, going to parties, driving miles to wait in bars for couples who didn't turn up, talking to men whose only purpose was to sleep with Mrs Bartell alone, changing their appearance to see whether they would be accepted, and investigating the homosexual side of the scene. They met more than 400 swingers, but by their own account, never actually had sex with anyone: if the moment of truth presented itself, they would awkwardly make their excuses and leave. Often, they would reveal that they were in fact academic researchers putting together an investigation of the scene, but other couples found it difficult to take this claim seriously, as it sounded too much like an elaborate excuse for taking part.

> Discreet, attractive couple 21 and 25 wish to meet couples and singles 21–35 for exciting and fun-loving adult relationships. Open-minded but not way out. No prejudices. Full length photo, address, and detailed letter assures same.
>
> Quoted in Bartell, *Group Sex*, *c.*1969–70

The typical male swinger in the Bartell's suburban sample read *Playboy* and aspired to its lifestyle, but was not, like the Californian orgiasts, some aesthetic bohemian disporting himself among the subtle shades of exotic plants and tanks of colourful tropical fish. Instead he and his wife were middle-class, white and conservative – not in itself that surprising since the survey drew heavily on evidence from the preponderantly white suburbs around Chicago. The women surveyed tended to be in their late twenties, the men in their early thirties. They had been married since the late 1950s or early 60s, and had two or three dependent children. Typically, they were middle managers, salesmen or housewives (together making up 78 per cent of respondents) and were the Republican offspring of blue-collar workers made good. Their ads often specified 'whites only'. Moreover, they stood against everything that long hair and hippies symbolised. When Bartell let his beard and hair grow as an experiment, the swingers shunned him. They might have adopted the sexual fashions of the period, but they stood resolutely against its political and cultural trends. To the Bartells, by their own account a 'hip' young couple from a university town, these people were an unappealing melange of all that was dull about middle America.

As well as being unfashionable, the average body type did not conform to the 'attractive' tag so often employed in the ads. The typical male was a slack-waisted, balding man of about 5' 10". Women averaged 5' 4" and if not exactly fat, had succumbed to the early ravages of middle-age spread. They were not enormously overweight but at the very least tended 'to be overendowed in the hips, thighs and stomach'. For all the advertised charms of big breasts, the women tended to be relatively flat-chested. Not that any of this was a problem for the Chicagoan swingers, since, like some lost tribe, their ideals of attractiveness were highly specific. The Bartells were continually told that one couple in particular were 'the most attractive couple in swinging', only to find when they did finally meet them that they were not that different from the others, and were in fact, 'very average, bland and what was once called "Aryan"'. By the standards of the swingers, though, who prized average-ness and familiarity, this was the height of sex appeal.[20]

How many swingers were there? Many of those investigating or promoting the scene as an element of the sexual revolution made wildly improbable estimates. Some said as many as 14 million. Others guessed as few as 70,000.[21] The Bartells reckoned that there were maybe 8,000 swingers in the Chicago area, and extrapolated from this a total US figure of between half and one million people, or 1 per cent of the population at most, a figure approximating to the circulation of swinging magazines.[22]

Swingers swung, Bartell and others argued, as an antidote to suburban boredom and alienation. In fact, expressions of discontent were never far from the surface at swinging house parties. Women would complain about husbands, home, housework and children, their irritation gradually blurring into 'an annoyed, generalized harangue'. Men would talk about sports, taxes and the threat to American life from Communism. Even allowing for the fact that the young and urbane Bartells were not exactly in tune with what they regarded as the rituals of the prematurely middle-aged, the impression of joylessness was overwhelming. Nothing ever satisfied these swingers, the Bartells concluded, and 'nothing was good and enjoyable'.[23] The homogenous interiors in which the parties took place reflected the dullness of swingers' talk, being made up of all the latest sixties mod cons: wall-to-wall carpeting in a beige-brown combination, plastic-covered furniture in the same earth tones, off-white or cream walls and curtains in a similar numbing shade of beige.

The function of swinging, from the Bartells' anthropological perspective, was not to break the bounds of middle-class morality or to liberate one's consciousness in the manner of the counterculture, but simply to try and combat feelings of isolation and frustration. Mate swapping or wife exchange of the kind the Bartells discovered in Chicago did have an analogue in less complex tribal societies, and that was done to form bonds of kinship or brotherhood. Among the Remer of Rwanda, or the Eskimos of north America, who had also been studied by Gilbert Bartell, mate exchange was a ritualised form of hospitality which implied a kind of 'blood brother' relationship between the giver and receiver. When men left their village or locality, bonds of this kind were vital in establishing a form of kinship in a harsh environment. For Bartell, the Chicago swingers were not unlike the Eskimos, adrift not in some snowy waste far from the support networks of blood relations, but lost in a beige suburban wilderness with only their immediate neighbours for company. Although the informal rules of swinging prevented emotional ties – sex was its sole and imperative aim – swinging did allow people to break out of their alienation and to establish friendship networks, however attenuated.[24] For all the men's aspirations to a *Playboy* lifestyle, many of the female swingers prized their contacts primarily as friends. One New Orleans couple reported that the answers to their ads came 'from the nicest people'. They were attractive, roughly the same age, with 'kids the age of ours, and they like to do everything we like to do. They told us about their house and it sounded just lovely!'

Another woman concurred: many of her contacts, she said, were her 'close friends'.[25] With its rule-bound rituals and suburban location, organised swinging was not that different from civic organisations like the PTA, a bowling league, or membership of the Shriners or Elks. Swinging, the Bartells concluded, was as American as apple pie.

Swinging for Britain

In Britain, by contrast, swinging was not nearly so organised or uniform. It was also probably more read about and fantasised over than actually done. There were certainly not as many swinging magazines in late-1960s Britain as there were in the US, but there were fifteen or sixteen which carried the ads.[26] Genuine British swingers also had to negotiate a less promising terrain than their American counterparts, weaving their way between the police, the pornographers and the prostitutes who advertised in contact mags. The company they kept in the personal column testified to the fact that swingers were still bracketed with those outside the law. The way the police in Britain investigated small-time magazines like *Exit* and *Way Out* while their American counterparts merely shrugged as their own swinging industry exploded, tells us everything about the differences between the two countries. That does not mean, however, that people in Britain didn't swing. The police investigation of *Exit* and *Way Out* in 1968 discovered 379 people who had corresponded through the magazine and more than 400 names on the papers' books. Some were fantasists, some were genuine, and some even appeared in a film, playing themselves.

The first inkling most Britons had that group sex might exist outside the pages of Roman history was when the Profumo affair erupted in 1963. The story of John Profumo, minister of war in the Conservative government, and his resignation after it emerged that he had lied to the House of Commons about having an extra-marital affair with the model and nightclub dancer Christine Keeler, is familiar enough. Profumo's resignation also drew both the Cold War and the low-rent world of West London drug dealers into the scandal as it was discovered that Keeler had also been involved with a Russian 'naval attaché' named Yevgeny Ivanov, to whom it was suggested that she might have inadvertently passed Britain's nuclear secrets, and with a small-time West Indian criminal named Lucky Gordon. This mixture of spying, drugs and illicit sex fatally undermined the Conservatives, who went on to lose the next general election.

M. 52. My husband and I wish to meet attractive couples with view to possible swapping and fun. We are 33 and 38 years old living on London/Essex borders. Please reply with photo.
Correspondent 19, 1969

The key features of the affair were the revelations of upper-class debauchery and the apparent hypocrisy of an establishment that preached high moral values for everyone but itself. The central figure, Christine Keeler, who worked at Murray's nightclub in Soho, had first got involved with Profumo through the offices of the society osteopath Stephen Ward. He made a habit of befriending young showgirls like Keeler and her friend Mandy Rice-Davies and drawing them into what was essentially an informal network of high-class call girls. Ward rented a house on the Cliveden Estate in Buckinghamshire, home of his friends the Astor family, where he held parties, often involving group sex, flagellation, voyeurism or any combination of the three. Christine Keeler, young, beautiful, game and apparently guileless, was his star, and became Ward's companion and confidante. During the course of the scandal, it emerged that both Profumo and Ivanov had attended swimming parties at Cliveden, and that Ward had basically been procuring women for his friends. In her memoirs, Keeler recalled being initiated into the world of sex parties by Ward. 'He had told me that they all began in a very respectable way', she wrote in 2002, 'there would be drinks, civilized conversation, dinner – and then, from what he said, everyone was at it like rabbits. Astonishingly, that was about right.' With Ward, she went to fancy Mayfair flats to watch couples having sex, and once attended a dinner party where there was a huge phallic table decoration smuggled in from Germany. At Ward's Cliveden cottage, 'It was always a posh crowd who arrived in chauffeur-driven Bentleys or Rolls-Royces' to enjoy the fun and games. It seemed to her then that 'having money dictated that you had group sex as often as you possibly could'.[27]

In 1963 the Profumo affair's heady mix of high-ish society, politicians, spies and slumming made the idea of group sex seem very far removed from the lives of most people. The scandal simply seemed to demonstrate that the British ruling class was irredeemably decadent, and that this sort of thing was done mainly by upper-class degenerates. A poll taken after the scandal showed that the British public believed that having mistresses was 'quite current' in high society.[28] But the idea of group sex did not remain at the margins of the popular imagination for long. Between 1963 and 1968, when the raid on *Exit* took place, the counterculture had emerged, and sexual experimentation moved away from its supposedly natural aristocratic habitat. In those five years, a whole generation of readers was introduced by papers like *IT* to the burgeoning sexual revolution. Unconventional sexual practices could no longer be said to be the preserve of the depraved upper classes – if, indeed, they ever had been.

When the Obscene Publications Squad confiscated the documents they found at the *Exit* offices in October 1968, they noted the names and addresses of more than 400 advertisers and collected more than 200 letters, sent for forwarding to the magazine's office. These revealed a cross-section of aspirant British swingers and were used to form the evidential case against Donelly and Mcguigan, namely that they had used the advertisements, as the indictment put it, 'to induce readers thereof to resort to the said advertisers for the purposes of fornication and of taking part in or witnessing other disgusting and immoral acts and exhibitions with intent thereby to debauch and corrupt public morals'.[29]

At the heart of the case was the accusation that *Exit* was mainly a vehicle for prostitutes, much like the earlier, and much more overt *Ladies' Directory*, a list of call girls which described their attributes to Soho punters in the late 1950s. One *Exit* advertiser, for example, 'Beautiful blonde model, 24, lovely figure' stated that she was looking for 'extra legal work to help with income', a wording that suggested a more than amateur interest in the swinging scene. When the police followed this up, they found that the woman who had placed the advertisement, the rather glamorous-sounding Suzanne Brunesdotter of respectable West Dulwich, was in fact not a young and curvaceous Scandinavian blonde but a 47-year-old British woman who claimed to have ambitions as a photographic model. Not surprisingly, they didn't believe her cover story and concluded that, 'undoubtedly she is a prostitute'. Another ad, 'Gentlemen sought by attractive lady, SAE, All answered (London)', also turned out to be from a suburban hooker in leafy Wimbledon. A certain K.176, by contrast, a 'Constant looker for the right female partner of under 35. Dr Zivago [sic] looks, 34 years, kind and understanding with large, steady equipment', looking to meet 'girls and couples under 35 for memorable sessions. Complete satisfaction and discretion assured. You may have tried others – try me and remember for quite a time', turned out to be an Asian businessman who said he was trying to attract women as a way of entertaining visiting colleagues who expected to have paid-for female company.

Out of nine advertisers interviewed by the police at the start of 1969, three were either prostitutes or were trying to procure them for other people. Others were fantasists of various kinds. As the Bartells had discovered, many of those new to the world of swinging used fantasy or pornography as a way into the scene as a preliminary to full involvement in sex. Some exchanged pornographic photos, either to explore the possibilities on offer without necessarily committing themselves, or to gain more instant gratification from looking at naked people. Others corresponded about sexual fantasies. One transvestite man, for example, in the character of 'Miss Jean Scott', wrote about various scenarios involving cross-dressing and bondage to another correspondent in Wales. Another ad, seemingly placed by a couple, turned out to be a vehicle for the husband's fantasies about lesbians.

'Lady, 32, seeks female who will make fun with me in front of my husband. Only genuine replies please', was actually placed by a 30-year-old man, a married office manager from south London who had also replied to ads in three other contact mags. He had seen *Way Out* and talked to his wife, with whom he had already made some amateur photographic pornography, about putting an ad in. She hadn't been that interested, but he had written one anyway, and got some replies. The whole point was not to actually meet lesbians, he told the police, but the ad was merely worded like that 'so as to get more interest'. It was no more than a 'kind of experiment'. His wife, he asserted, 'would never do anything like that . . .' but he had invited some people to meet them and replied in his wife's name. After being questioned he said, 'I no longer do this', and swore that he had torn up all the letters except one that had come from a woman in the Canary Islands. The police, on the hunt for organised prostitution of any kind in order to prove their case against *Exit*, remained suspicious.

This man wasn't the only advertiser to adopt a fantasy persona. There was, for example, the 54-year-old male advertising executive who posed as a 'long-haired, full-bosomed, sensitive, 28 years Oriental girl, long unawakened after too long in private schools', looking for 'shy, submissive girls (like I once was) who are still pondering and seeking how to develop their secret wishes/tastes/talents for richer excitement'. He claimed to have done this to widen his appeal, but confessed he hadn't actually met anyone because all those who responded sounded like prostitutes. A 25-year-old husband from Middlesex – 'Educated married couple, 26, wish to meet same, or solo females under 50, who are DIY enthusiasts. Will exchange correspondence, photos, books, etc. We want to be viewed (no more than that) by a selected few only' – claimed that the ads he placed were 'only a phase I'm going through'. '[I] didn't want to meet anybody else really', he said, 'I just wanted to exchange experiences in letters.' Nevertheless he did have a couple of photos sent by other advertisers of their wives who, as the police noted, were 'both in the nude'.[30]

All these advertisers strenuously denied ever doing anything more than fantasising with their pen pals. Of course, they were unlikely to say anything else when confronted at their homes by two detectives from Scotland Yard. And even if they had met anyone and had sex with them, they wouldn't have been guilty of any crime. The reason they were being harassed was because the police needed evidence that *Exit* was commonly used by prostitutes. In fact, they found hardly any evidence which suggested that this was the case. In the course of their enquiries, though, the police did discover a few genuine swingers on the American model.

One ad in particular demonstrates the peculiar twists and turns of the swinging scene. The ad itself, 'Ann, 23, docile and beautiful, turned on, invites versatile girls (with or without attractive partners) to come and complete our happiness (London)', turned out to have been placed by a TV executive named Elkan Allan, a producer for Associated Rediffusion and the inventor of the hit pop-music show *Ready Steady Go!* In 1967, Allan had used the personal columns of *The Times*, the *New Statesman, Evening Standard* and *IT* to find subjects for his film *Love in Our Time*, a survey of contemporary sexual attitudes, and his latest ad in *Exit*, he said, was designed to attract homosexuals of both sexes, about whom he was making a new film. Although this ad might look ambiguous, he told the police, his earlier research had brought real swingers into the full glare of publicity, and shown that such things did exist behind the doors of the most respectable British homes.

Allan's film, *Love in Our Time*, featured a real couple who had arranged some of their wife swapping activities through *Exit*. Both them fitted the model of swinging so painstakingly outlined in the American research of Gilbert Bartell. Yvonne was thirty-five, Andre was forty-five. They lived in a semi-detached house on the edge of an English village and were happily married with children. The thought of wife swapping had never even occurred to either of them until one of Andre's business contacts asked him if he'd like to sleep with his wife. Andre was amazed, but intrigued, and during the course of several conversations came round to the idea. Yvonne was reluctant at first, but agreed to go and have dinner with the other couple in a hotel. There, they got pleasantly drunk and more or less spontaneously retreated to a convenient bedroom. After initial fumbling, Yvonne remembered thinking, as they exchanged partners, 'Well, we'd better go the whole way now'. She was surprised by her lack of jealousy and found that it reinvigorated her sex life with her husband. Both saw wife swapping not as something 'way out', or as a substitute for marital sex, but as a mutual pursuit, a kind of hobby that could be pursued together, and as a way of making their marriage even better. It was a safety valve, a kind of infidelity so ritualised that it was rendered harmless.[31]

For Allan, couples like Andre and Yvonne represented the real sexual revolution. They showed that 'the outer reaches of sexual behaviour had become nearer', spreading beyond the counterculture and into the lives of conventional middle-class men and women.[32] Some of the letters confiscated from *Exit* seemed to bear out this impression. Amidst the fantasies of corporal punishment and rubber wear, and the enticing ads of 'housewives' with time on their hands, those not included in the politics of the counter-culture tried to find each other. Many of the letters collected from the *Exit* offices by the police are written in the same warm, almost caring tone that the Bartells found to be characteristic of middle-class swingers in the US. Many were from 'Reasonably circumstanced, professional middle class folk', such as Michael L., the 50-year-old intellectual and professional type with a petite 32-year-old wife with whom he had had many 'pleasant experiences with foursome arrangements which we can enjoy at various levels of participation'. Letter-writers were often, just like Andre and Yvonne, at pains to point out their ordinariness. Swinging was fine, two *Exit* advertisers said, but 'we don't make a compulsive habit of it

> Where can my husband and I find another happily married couple or couples under 35 in the North Staffs area, for broadminded friendship. Interested and well equipped for photography. We enjoy life and wish to share with others of similar tastes. Photograph please, draped or undraped. This is our very first advert.
>
> *Correspondent* 19, 1969

– just when people are interesting and have something spirited and rewarding to contribute'.[33] These more genuine advertisers liked 'happy people who enjoy life and love variety and people', and were themselves well educated, 'polished with a marked sense of humour' and had 'no rough corners or kinks', but did frequently possess 'a very healthy sexual appetite which must be satisfied soon or I fear I may bust!'[34] For Michael, while abhorring intolerance, it was nevertheless imperative to 'insist on standards and intuitive decency'.

The truth about wife swapping in Britain is that amidst all the fantasies it engendered it did actually happen, and that *Exit*'s ads helped it, and many other kinds of sex, take place – whether paid for or not. Swinging was less organised than in the US, and was mixed in with a whole slew of other sexual identities and habits, but was nevertheless one way of putting the ideology of sexual revolution into some kind of practice. Many welcomed swinging, including authoritative figures like the veteran sex radical and doctor Eustace Chesser, who thought that the rebellion against conventional morals represented by couples like Yvonne and Andre broke down repression and would allow other less adventurous spirits to live a more balanced and less anxious life. Small rebellions like theirs, however ambivalent, could change the mainstream for ever. The American writer Edward M. Brecher, in his study of sex, also agreed that swinging might be therapeutic for those suffering from the inheritance of 'Victorian' sexual repressions.[35]

Yet in spite of these endorsements, and all their attempts at normality, swingers and the media through which they made contact did not get a good press. In part, this was because, as the response of the police to *IT* and *Exit* showed, much of what passed for sexual revolution in Britain remained on the edges of legality. The popular verdict was equally cautious and conservative. The readers of the *Sunday People*, asked to sit in judgement on Allan's *Love in Our Time*, concluded that 'they ought to call it LUST in our time'. They felt that even this relatively cautious film should not have been made, and they argued that its subjects were 'a menace to decent society'. Wife swappers were no better than pimps, the *People*'s star letter argued. 'Is not a man who barters his wife in exchange for the sexual use of another woman equally as criminal?'[36]

The problem was that the rhetoric of sexual revolution which informed the counterculture of the late 1960s concealed a deep ambivalence, even in those who participated fully in it. As the underground editor Richard Neville put it, as soon as it had been announced at the end of the sixties, the sexual revolution had become a cliché, declared annually with the coming of spring. Its tempting and various delights, as depicted on the screen or in the papers, hardly ever reached real life, and when they did so, it was in the compromised form of ambiguous small ads, feeble plays like *Oh! Calcutta*, or the ample frames of podgy suburban swingers. Neville discovered that even in 1970 it was still impossible for an unmarried couple to book a double room at Claridge's hotel in London, get a chalet at a holiday camp or reserve a double cabin on a P&O liner.[37] As the oral historian and sixties participant Jonathon Green puts it, the sexual revolution both succeeded and failed. It raised hopes and expanded horizons, but left most people exactly as they had been before.[38] The problem with swinging, wife swapping and all the rest was that its advocates expected too much from it: personal liberation, cultural change, the overthrow of 'Victorian' morality, even the beginning of a new world. The American sex researcher John Simon rightly pointed out in 1970 that the most outlandish aspects of modern sex, such as swinging, were 'symptomatic of our current overloading of the sexual, making it stand for more than it can really be'.[39]

Amidst all this confusion, one of the successes of the counterculture, one that was to catch on as a medium for love, sex and adventure with increasing force over the following twenty years, remained relatively unnoticed: the small ad. Ads were crucial to the self-identity of the counterculture, and as a result they carried on the long tradition of personal advertising as a subversive medium. This sense of continued defiance among the classifieds was reinforced by the attacks of the police and courts on their wilder outposts. However, the long drawn out and ultimately successful prosecutions of *IT* (1969–72) and *Exit* (1968–72) for carrying gay contact ads turned out to be no more than a pyrrhic victory for the authorities. Going right up to the House of Lords in order to finish off a small-timer like Edward Donelly was worse than breaking a butterfly on a wheel; it made the police and Home Office look ridiculous.

Couple in 20s would like to meet other couples in 20s for swapping parties, single girls welcome. Can accommodate, would travel reasonable distance. Frank reply. Photo please.

Correspondent 19, 1969

As it turned out, these cases were the last of the many

legal persecutions of lonely hearts, homosexuals and swingers that dated back to the beginnings of advertising itself. It wasn't only the excesses of the police that helped the personal ad eventually escape the shackles of the law, though. By the early 1970s, the new techniques of media production pioneered by the counterculture had gone mainstream, appearing on every bookstall in colour supplements and women's magazines, and it was not long before underground classifieds and lonely hearts, both gay and straight, swinging and square, became staple features of ordinary journalism. *Time Out*, by 1971 no longer a badly printed poster-sized underground news sheet but now in its familiar magazine format, began in that year to print a few lonely hearts ads as a constituent part of the magazine. Swingers, hippies and countercultural types rubbed shoulders in *Time Out*'s early personals. By September 1971, the 'Two married couples, Surrey area', looking to meet other couples for 'very swinging evenings', could do so without a great deal of trepidation.[40]

Epilogue

The Internet, or, This Chapter Will Shortly Be Out of Date

JDate, Plentyoffish, *Guardian* Soulmates, Meetic, Match.com, Gaydar, GaydarGirls, Friends Reunited Dating TM, Mysinglefriend®, Illicit Encounters, NewFriends4U, Dating Direct, Tummy Butterflies, Shaadi.com, Love Horse, Loopylove, Truedate, Ivory Towers, Love and Friends . . . These are only a few of the many dating sites which now exist to cater for those in the UK looking for love, sex, partnership and even marriage. Above all, the internet has brought speed and immediacy to the world of the personals. Love and courtship is now smarter and faster. But is it better? Is it really that different? In short, has the internet transformed our social and romantic lives?

You could say that the internet merely accelerates processes which, when people had to rely on print and the postal service, just took longer to achieve. Like the personal column, the correspondence club or the introduction agency, the internet caters to the need to reach out, to create communities and contacts beyond the reach of familial authority and sometimes out of sight of the law. But while the users of the personal column hid behind often elaborate codes, now, self-revelation is the key. If you're under thirty and you don't have an internet profile, a MySpace account, a blog, a Second Life, if you can't be Googled or Facebooked, then you barely exist. Being networked in this way is a key sign of participation in a social life. Without an internet profile, how can you participate in what the sociologist Manuel Castells calls the 'network society' in which social existence is defined mainly by the networks to which you belong, and by how you maintain contact with the others in that network?[1] Unlike the personal column, where disguise was frequently essential, the internet seems to compel us to tell all – or at least edited highlights – about ourselves, to render up our experience for observation, to detail everything to the readers of our blog. Never before have we been so willing to place ourselves under scrutiny.

In the mid-1990s, when the internet started to become more accessible in Britain and America, high hopes were attached to it. Many writers and academics began to argue that it was a kind of new frontier, a place where a new kind of community and a new kind of self would develop. The closest analogy was the invention of print in the fifteenth century. Just as that had eventually undermined existing religious orthodoxies and created a whole new democratic public for the press and pamphlet (not to mention the advertisement), so in the internet age new ways of thinking would emerge, a new kind of radical public would develop dedicated to rational debate and pushing forward the bounds of human knowledge. Early internet guru Manuel Castells even compared it to the invention of the alphabet in ancient Greece. Just as that had encouraged the rise of abstract thought, the internet, with its integration of the written, the oral and the audio-visual, would profoundly change the nature of human communication.[2]

Our personal interactions would also be transformed. We

would live cyberlives, liberated not only from the constraints of time and place, but also from our earth-bound bodies. It was envisaged that the chatroom would not be a forum for threatening perverts, as a series of subsequent child pornography and stalking scandals later suggested, but a kind of village square where people of like minds could get together and re-establish the fragile bonds of community. The characteristic feature of cyberculture, as it was called at the end of the 1990s, was supposed to be the separation of real life (RL) and online life. It was assumed that these would be incompatible and fundamentally different. This would be nowhere more obvious than in the realm of intimacy, love and sex. The internet and its associated technologies would allow us to transcend the human body and enter a new world of cyborg sexuality. We would meet and enter relationships online, even have sex online, all without meeting the other person. These interactions would be so all-consuming that we would have to be wary of these relationships taking us over. It was proposed that online life could be so attractive, and the possibility of creating multiple selves so seductive, that we might even develop personality disorders.[3]

These speculations were the academic equivalent of the dot.com boom. Just as that economic bubble relied on a dramatic overconfidence about what the internet was capable of in the realm of commerce, sociologists, cybergurus and assorted other commentators lined up to tell us that human life and consciousness would never be the same again. The internet and its related technologies would ensure that soon we might even become cyborgs, interacting directly with machines wired into our bodies. This was the internet as in

The Matrix, a world in which cybersex 'heralds the disappearance of the human–machine interface', a merging which would destroy our existing notion of self by throwing the 'one-time individual into a pulsing network of switches'. The 'natural' self would disappear, along with 'natural' bodies and sexualities, to be replaced by mechanical and psychotropic technologies, by 'drugs, trance and dance possession; androgyny, hermaphroditism and transsexualism . . . paraphilia [and] body engineering'.[4]

Even if we discount this kind of revolutionary rhetoric, it is nevertheless true that people have developed relationships that are mainly or exclusively online. One study done in the last decade showed that many respondents found these online relationships much more fulfilling and open than their real-life ones. The immediacy of email or instant messaging meant that they were able to reveal much more to their online friends and lovers than they were to those with whom they shared their lives. Distance, it seemed, lent a great deal of enchantment to the view. These friendships were, according to the sociologist Aaron Ben Ze'ev, a distinctively new type of personal relationship, one that offered what he calls 'intimate closeness at a distance'. He found that online friends were much more revealing and honest than they were in real life. This was partly because email and the internet liberated users from the things that held them back in ordinary social interactions. You were no longer influenced by what someone looked like, their manner, what they wore, or by the many signs and tics which indicated their class or social standing. These relationships were not only more based in the imagination, but were also more egalitarian, Ben Ze'ev concluded. They were, in effect, a 'new type of personal relationship'.[5]

Online lives and relationships have encouraged fears that people, especially the young, spend far too much time in front of computers, working on virtual relationships and neglecting real ones. Newspaper commentators, particularly in the period of Web 1.0 that preceded the burst of the dot.com bubble, have churned out stories of internet zombies, uber-nerds who rarely left their favourite chatroom or networking site. But has the internet actually altered personal relationships in this way? Those who have studied actual internet use say that it hasn't. Instead of the internet leading to social isolation or online absorption, as the early 'new frontier'/Web 1.0-type writers suggested, it has in fact tended to increase offline networking and social interactions. Use of email and the internet actually correlates with a much wider social life and absorption in social networks. Instead of Web 1.0, in which online life was thought to replace real interactions, we now inhabit the world of Web 2.0, in which social networks such as MySpace and user-generated content like YouTube or blogging dominate the Web. According to recent studies, these sites are used to bolster and encourage real-world social networks, not to replace them. College students use Facebook to arrange dates, MySpace or Bebo users go over what happened at school that day, while internet dating has never been more popular. For all its revolutionary potential, the internet has merely accelerated long-standing social trends which have encouraged the dispersal of social groups and more individualistic types of communication.[6]

This is nowhere more obvious than in the world of online

dating and romance. Ever since the seventeenth century, advertising for love has been accused of being cold and unromantic, calculating and even just plain sad, in spite of the fact that large numbers of people actually did it. The same suspicions still surround internet dating, but more people than ever use it to find friendship and romance. The inheritors of the legacy left by the *Link*, the Universal Correspondence Club and the Marriage Bureau are numerous. Collectively, the leading sites such as Match.com, Dating Direct and French site Meetic, claim more than 45 million members between them in more than 240 countries.[7] Meetic has 22 million members in seventeen countries, while Match.com claims over 200,000 new users a month. In May 2007, dating sites received 6.4 million unique visitors in Britain alone.[8]

The more direct sensibility of internet dating has also crossed over into other areas of modern life. Speed dating, which sacrifices romance for convenience, has never been more popular, while dating guides which offer rigid rules for self-presentation drawn from marketing theory sell in their thousands. As the French journalist Agnès Poirier has pointed out, the language of consumerism and economics translates effortlessly to the new realm of internet romance. It is, she suggests, a simple matter of supply and demand: pre-select candidates, test sales pitch, draw a shortlist, have a face-to-face interview, hire on the spot, enjoy casual sex, and 'dismiss without notice, Voila – a case of ultra-liberalism meets romance'.[9]

The epitome of this kind of accelerated, targeted dating is the gay men's website Gaydar, established in 1999, and now with over 4 million registered users in twenty-three countries, more than a million of them in Britain. Although it can be used to find long-term relationships or friendships of all kinds, the dominant way of using Gaydar (slogan: 'What you want, when you want it') is to find no-strings sex. Historically, gay men have tended to pride themselves on rejecting the paraphernalia of heterosexual romance, preferring instead the greater honesty of getting straight to the point. Gaydar crystallises this sensibility into a series of questions in which users specify their sexual preferences including penis size, role (active, passive, versatile), body hair and attire. 'It's literally as easy as ordering in a pizza', one user told the *Guardian* in 2007.[10] GaydarGirls, an exact copy of the men's site by the same company with more than 245,000 members and 8,000 new ones each month, 90 per cent of whom are in Britain, is also said to have transformed lesbian attitudes to casual sex. Thanks in part to Gaydar, the lesbian scene is said to be more 'cruisy', and more similar to the world of gay men than ever before. According to Gaydar's critics, cruising for sex is now no longer an exciting encounter with the unknown that requires adaptability, give and take, and a kind of communal and friendly in-this-together kind of feeling. Moreover, Gaydar and the internet have tended to accelerate the privatisation of gay life more generally, restricting it to the home, even to the detriment of gay bars and social spaces. For Stephen Maddison, a cultural studies academic, the world of Gaydar has changed cruising into a business, 'turning adventure into a sexual McDonald's'.[11]

Trends in the world of gay dating are not isolated from broader currents, and there are many examples of straight men and women employing exactly similar tactics. According to one 2004 survey carried out by Friends Reunited, the most successful key words in any internet profile were those which stressed the physical, such as 'sensual, wild, tactile and sexy'.[12] There are also sites specifically devoted to arranging affairs between the married and disenchanted, the main ones being the appropriately named Illicit Encounters (mainly for men) and the cutesy-sounding Tummy Butterflies for women. Research carried out by those sites suggested that more than a third of married women between twenty and sixty 'already have a secret affair very much in mind'.[13] Some of these women may end up as one of the familiar features of the more mature straight scene: the legendary POWs or 'Predatory Older Women', successful professionals of a certain age in Armani suits and expensive cars who trawl the dating sites looking not for relationships but for what one man describes as 'uncomplicated sex three or four times a month'.[14]

In spite of this evidence, some researchers, including one from the University of Bath who has worked as a consultant for Match.com, have argued that, paradoxically, romance is actually making a comeback on the net. Psychologist Jeff Gavin's 2005 survey of 229 users showed that 94 per cent of respondents had met their 'most significant online relationship' more than once, and that when relationships took place, they lasted on average seven months, which compared favourably with other kinds of introduction. Moreover, 18 per cent of the relationships established (we are not told what proportion of total contacts this was) lasted for more than a year, which might be regarded as either a low or high figure, depending on your perspective. The point is that these ambiguous figures were used to demonstrate that 'old-fashioned romance isn't dead'.[15]

However, the popularity of internet dating revealed in surveys like this tends not to demonstrate conclusively that real romance is either vital or moribund, but that there is a paradox in modern attitudes to dating and love. While we continue to believe in the power of romance as an idea, and cling to the hope that all will one day end in hearts and flowers, the way we use the internet does seem to suggest a more calculating approach to love and sex. One of the concerns about Web 2.0 is that it encourages a narrowing of horizons, an arena in which only the like-minded ever talk to or see each other. As one recent critic of Web 2.0 argues, social networking sites of all kinds do not generate a healthy culture of rational debate and dissent, a shattering of the self as promised by the web gurus of the 1990s. Instead 'people of like minds congregate to confirm what they want'.[16] The detailed profiles which internet dating employs act in a similar way, requiring readers to specify preferences and their own characteristics even without the space for extensive self-description. The question remains: has widespread internet use made us focused about our wants, and cynical about love, as earlier critics of advertising for romance always claimed it would? Has it made us blind to the unexpected, and encouraged us in a narrow search for what we already like and know? The British still flock to films like *Love Actually*, with its celebration of love's power, but at the same time, we seem never to have been more calculating about the costs and benefits of romance.

The feeling that we want to believe in romance, but somewhat against our better judgement, is one that is perhaps spreading in the contemporary world. Social life, including love, sex and romance, have been changed in myriad ways, and this is reflected in, rather than inspired by, patterns of internet use. Marriage rates are falling all over the world, especially in Britain and Europe, but, as the historian Stephanie Coontz points out, this has been accompanied by an increasing reverence for the idea of romantic love.[17] Resulting paradoxes abound. While two-thirds of British people canvassed in 2007 saw little difference between marriage and cohabitation, weddings have become bigger than ever, with £20,000 being the average amount spent.[18]

A few years ago, the gnomic Italian philosopher and novelist Umberto Eco summed up the situation when he argued that the contemporary paradox of love epitomised the modern condition. Love was like all those other stories we had been telling ourselves in Western society, stories of endless progress, liberation and rationality, none of which we really believed in any longer. Like romance, they had all been trampled on once too often. 'One can no longer say, "I love you madly" because Barbara Cartland has already said it', argued Eco. 'Instead, we can only say to our beloved, "as Barbara Cartland would put it, I love you madly".'[19] Like all the other articles of modern liberal faith, the idea of romantic love had become tarnished through repetition and overuse and was no longer useful, other than as an ironic return of an earlier belief. More recently, Eco's suspicion has been echoed by many other commentators. As a senior counsellor from Relate, the successor of the National Marriage Guidance Council, put it in 2006, many people expect less from love these days, and still less from marriage. 'People are much more realistic about marriage these days', she said. 'We've all grown up a bit, we're a bit more emotionally intelligent than we were. We know marriages are not uniformly romantic and happy.'[20]

One reason for this clear-eyed approach to romance, which can be found on countless internet sites, may lie in the fact that the online dating market is highly segregated by age. Young people (i.e. under twenty-five) who think nothing of meeting or hooking up via MySpace or Facebook tend to baulk at using a dating site like Guardian Soulmates (85,000 active members). This means that dating sites like Soulmates tend to be (on average) for those in their thirties – people who know better than to succumb at first glance to hearts and flowers, or at least think they do. This is true across Europe, where the average age of Meetic users in France is thirty-two, and in Spain thirty-five.[21] The fact that long-term partnership, and especially marriage, is now generally deferred in the West until the late twenties or early thirties, when financial and job security have been achieved, also means that those on the dating market in general are now in an older age group than they have ever been. Older might not mean wiser, but it does tend to offer perspective. The young, who generally don't use dating sites, have a different attitude to romance, if internet surveys can be trusted. One 2004 survey conducted by researchers Future Laboratory for Match.com showed that, in spite of their reputation for promiscuity, those under thirty 'felt incredibly strongly about fidelity and monogamy and the need to meet that one person, fall in love with them and live with them'. Those between thirty-four and forty-five, on the other hand, were less bothered by infidelity and were cynical about monogamy, preferring cohabitation to marriage.[22]

All the evidence suggests that the internet has not necessarily revolutionised intimacy or personal identity, but has emphasised other contemporary trends, not least that of economic independence and its corollary, the need to sell oneself – to be 'flexible' – in response to a variety of social and economic pressures. The widespread scepticism about the validity of marriage is also reflected in the age-segregated dating market. If we think that we've got a functional attitude to love, it's only because, as Umberto Eco sagely pointed out, we're cynical – or sceptical – about a lot of other things.

In that respect, the internet hasn't transformed social life so much as continued and accelerated the trends once pioneered by the likes of Alfred Barrett and his ill-fated *Link*. The benefits of anonymity and the opportunism involved in making use of new media is still a way of getting beyond traditional types of authority, usually that of the family. Just as those women who used matrimonial advertising in the 1820s, or those seeking pals a century later, were bypassing traditional sources of parental or social authority and asserting their right to make their own choices, so are the teenage users of MySpace, whether arranging parties, mass public pillow fights, or hook-ups.

What *is* different about Web 2.0, as opposed to its ancestor the personal column, is that self-revelation is now compulsory. We haven't transcended ourselves, as some writers thought we would, but become ever more ourselves. The directness of email and instant messaging encourages self-revelation, spontaneity and an easy assumption of intimacy. At the same time, on Web 2.0 we seek out exactly what we want, we rarely depart from our personal preferences, we look only at our favourites or fans. Far from giving us multiple selves, the internet as it is now merely allows us to examine the one we've already got ad nauseam, to parade it continually to a relatively small circle of like minds. As one Web 2.0 guru concedes, on the internet everyone will be famous to fifteen people.[23]

The internet, like the *Link*, the lonely soldiers, the correspondence club and the matrimonial ad, looks both ways, forward and back. The ambiguity of the small ad and its successors has allowed people to experiment with new freedoms, to assert their competence and independence, to remain 'refined' while simultaneously being 'sporty'. At the same time, these media have offered the hope of giving us the things we have always wanted – work, material goods, love, marriage. Alfred Barrett of *Link* fame recognised this in 1916. The old order of love, romance and respectability had given way to something difficult to define, yet something that was undoubtedly 'entirely new and subversive'. The modern girl was more than a match for her brother, Barrett said, but although she was now resourceful and self-reliant, with a 'healthy understanding of life', that did not necessarily mean the end of sentiment. Innovators like Barrett often feel the need to reassure, and he felt certain that somewhere along the path of progress 'the eternal He' would be waiting for even the most advanced modern woman. She was merely taking a more interesting route to her destination. After all, a kiss was still a kiss, and 'men and maidens', not to mention artistic young men and their lonely soldiers, would 'still walk in couples in the gloaming'.[24]

Acknowledgements

Thanks to the librarians and staff of the National Archives Kew, the British Library St Pancras and Colindale, Mass Observation at the University of Sussex, John Rylands Library University of Manchester, Manchester Central Library, University of London Library Senate House, the History of Advertising Trust, the Women's Library and Birkbeck College. To my agent, Charlie Viney for showing a lot of faith in the project, and to Nigel Wilcockson, Emily Rhodes, Louise Campbell and everyone at Random House. Also to Richard Johnson, Anne Charvet and Sarah Child, who offered editorial advice and contacts. For their generosity in providing me with useful references and sources, many thanks especially to Helen Berry, and also to Peter Bailey, Matt Cook, Matt Houlbrook and Vincent Quinn. Thanks to all my family and friends, especially Micah Buis for his insightful and diplomatic analysis of the first draft, to Belete Holt-Fente for always being so positive about the book (sorry I couldn't make it 33 per cent funnier), Gerry Gunning, Julie-Marie Strange, Chris Waters, James Vernon, Teresa Neil, Ishwar Maharaj, Robert Maidens, Jon Atkin, Emma Duggan, Frank Geary, Stephen Legg, Charles Watkins and my colleagues in the School of History, University of Nottingham. Thanks also to students from 'Gender, Sex and Society in 20th Century Britain', 'Love and Intimacy in Anglo-American Culture', 'The Rule of Freedom' and 'Rethinking the Victorians'. Finally, and most importantly, eternal gratitude to my family for making it possible for me to write this book.

Parts of Chapters 1 and 2 were first published as 'Sporty Girls and Artistic Boys: Friendship, Illicit Sex, and the British Companionship Advertisement 1913–1928', *Journal of the History of Sexuality* 11, 3, pp. 457–82.

Parts of Chapters 3, 5 and 6 were first published as 'Peril in the Personals: The Pleasures and Dangers of Classified Advertising in Early 20th Century Britain', *Media History* 10 (2004), pp. 3–17, and 'Saucy Stories: Pornography, Sexology and the Marketing of Sexual Knowledge in Britain *c.* 1918–1970', *Social History* 29 (2004), pp. 465–87. I am grateful for permission to reproduce this material. See www.informaworld.com.

Illustration acknowledgements:

p. 13 photograph from *Daily Mirror*, 22 April 1921, p. 9 © British Library Board. All Rights Reserved (shelfmark MLD4)

p. 37 advertisement for Phyllis Monkman from *Pearson's Weekly*, 8 July 1916, p. 16 © British Library Board. All Rights Reserved (shelfmark LD119)

p. 47 *Daily Mirror*, 27 December 1921, p. 9 © British Library Board. All Rights Reserved (shelfmark MLD4)

p. 68 *Daily Mirror*, 15 December 1925, p. 1 © British Library Board. All Rights Reserved (shelfmark MLD4)

p. 90 1920s postcard © Mary Evans Picture Library

p. 111 *Ballyhoo*, October 1933 cover © British Library Board. All Rights Reserved (shelfmark PP 6383ckb). By kind permission of the publisher Random House Inc.

p. 134 article by David Mace from *John Bull*, 20 March 1948, p. 5 © British Library Board. All Rights Reserved (shelfmark LD116)

p. 150 classified pages from *Time Out* London, 24–30 December 1971, issue number 97. Reproduced with kind permission of Time Out Group Ltd

Notes

Introduction

1. 'Seeking Romance: GSOH and Web 2.0 Compatibility Essential', *Guardian*, 12 July 2007; 'Record Users for Bebo and Facebook', *Guardian*, 19 May 2008.
2. This was known as 'The Pyes of Salisbury'. See T. R. Nevett, *Advertising in Britain, A History* (London, 1982), p. 8.
3. I am very grateful to Helen Berry for information on this subject. See Helen Berry, *Gender, Society and Print Culture in Late-Stuart England: The Cultural World of the Athenian Mercury* (Aldershot, 2003).
4. Anonymous cutting (1777) in Anon., *Matrimonial Advertisements*, Private Collection, *c.* 1740–1859, British Library.
5. In this case, her judgement was awry, as Mary Moore's future husband turned out to be the murderer William Corder. See J. Curtis, *An Authentic and Faithful History of the Mysterious Murder of Maria Marten* . . . (London, 1828), p. 92.

Chapter 1

1. Indictment against Barrett, Smith, Smyth and Birks, cited in CID Report, 14 June 1921, *The Link, Corrupting Public Morals*, National Archives Kew (hereafter TNA) MEPO 3/283.
2. *Daily Telegraph*, 8 June 1921.
3. Vernon to Walter Birks, 1 December 1919, TNA MEPO 3/283.
4. William Smyth to Birks, 21 October 1920, TNA MEPO 3/283.
5. CID Report, 18 April 1921, TNA MEPO 3/283.

6. *Link*, March 1921, p. 4.
7. CID Report, 23 May 1921; 30 May 1921, TNA MEPO 3/283. *Link*, March 1921, p. 1.
8. *Link*, March 1921, p. 1.
9. *Link*, November 1916, p. 1.
10. *News of the World*, 8 May 1921.
11. *Link*, November 1919; September 1920, p.1.
12. *Link*, September 1920, p. 1.
13. *Link*, September 1920, p. 1.
14. *Link*, December 1918, p. 1.
15. *Link*, November 1919, p. 1.
16. *Daily Telegraph*, 9 June 1921.
17. R. Andom, *The Strange Adventures of Roger Wilkins and Other Stories* (London, 1895), dedication.
18. CID Report, 18 April 1921, TNA MEPO 3/283.
19. See, on this, George Robb, 'The Way of All Flesh: Degeneration, Eugenics, and the Gospel of Free Love', *Journal of the History of Sexuality*, 6, 4 (1996): pp. 589–601.
20. *The Adult: The Journal of Sex*, 2, 1 (February 1898), back cover.
21. *T. P.'s Weekly*, 27 February 1915, p. 220.
22. *T. P.'s Weekly*, 12 February 1916, p. 166.
23. *T. P.'s Weekly*, 2 January 1914, p. 26.
24. *T. P.'s Weekly*, 9 January 1914, p. 124.
25. *T. P.'s Weekly*, 20 March 1915, p. 291.
26. *Daily Telegraph*, 11 June 1921.

CHAPTER 2

1. *Daily Express*, 4 March 1915, p. 2.
2. Cpl Fred Woods to *Express*, 8 March 1915, quoted in *Daily Express*, 13 March 1915.
3. Susan R. Grayzel 'Mothers, Marraines and Prostitutes: Morale

and Morality in First World War France', *International History Review*, 19, 1 (1997): pp. 66–82; Grayzel, *Women's Identities at War: Gender, Motherhood and Politics in Britain and France During the First World War* (Chapel Hill, NC, 1999).

4. Grayzel, 'Mothers, Marraines', pp. 70–75.
5. Magnus Hirschfeld, *The Sexual History of the Great War* (New York, 1934), p. 72.
6. 'Friends in Council', *T. P.'s Weekly*, 5 February 1916, p. 143.
7. *T. P.'s Weekly*, 12 February 1916, p. 166.
8. *T. P.'s Weekly*, February 1916, p. 191; *Link*, October 1918, p. 10; November 1918, p. 11; December 1919.
9. S. P. B. Mais, *April's Lonely Soldier* (London, 1916), p. 11. See also May Aldington, *Love Letters to a Soldier* (London, 1915). The *Times Literary Supplement* praised both novels as pleasant and unremarkable reading for railway journeys. *TLS*, 21 September 1916, p. 452; 17 August 1916, p. 395.
10. Mais, *April's Lonely Soldier*, p. 11.
11. T. P. Hobbins, Capt R. E., to OC 50th Batt, enc. to Col. W. Price, Director, Postal Services, BEF, 6 February 1915, *Lonely Soldier Correspondence*, TNA HO 139/32.
12. G. E. P. Murray [Sec of GPO] to Sir Stanley Buckmaster, 25 March 1915, *Lonely Soldier Correspondence*, TNA HO 139/32.
13. D-Notice 406, 24 May 1916, *Lonely Soldier Correspondence*, TNA HO 139/32.
14. J. Mullaney to *People*, 2 October 1916, *Lonely Soldier Correspondence*, TNA HO 139/32.
15. 'Who Will Marry Phyllis Monkman? A Chance for Single Men', *Pearson's Weekly*, 8 July 1916, p. 67.
16. 'Who Will Marry Phyllis Monkman? *Pearson's Weekly*, 29 July 1916, p. 166.
17. *Pearson's Weekly*, 12 August 1916, p. 166.
18. H. Knox-Swan of Press Bureau, 10 June 1916, *Lonely Soldier Correspondence*, TNA HO 139/32.

19. General Routine Orders, 13 April 1916. Adjutant General's Branch 1503 Correspondence with Strangers, *Lonely Soldier Correspondence*, TNA HO 139/32.
20. *Daily Chronicle*, quoted in *Link*, October 1919; *Link*, January 1918, p. 1.
21. *Daily Express*, 8–31 July 1924. Some of these were little different from those which had convicted Barrett. For example the 'broad minded' bachelor seeking a 'male chum evenings and week-ends'. *Daily Express*, 31 July 1924, p. 11.
22. Vero Garratt, 'Youth and Marriage', *English Review* (May 1923): pp. 473–79, p. 477.

Chapter 3

1. William Tylar, *The Spirit of Irene Speaks* (Bournemouth, 1923).
2. 'Crime and Motive . . . Sir Basil Thomson's Suggestions', *The Times*, 30 December 1921, p. 9.
3. Tylar, *Spirit of Irene*, p. 64.
4. W. Lloyd Woodland, *The Trial of Thomas Henry Allaway* (London, 1929), p. 29.
5. Nevett, *Advertising in Britain*, pp. 114–15.
6. Sir Arthur Conan Doyle, 'The Red-Headed League', in *The Adventures of Sherlock Holmes* (London, 1892), pp. 177–90, p. 178.
7. *Link*, July 1916, p. 2.
8. Laura Hutton, *The Single Woman and Her Emotional Problems* (Baltimore, 1935).
9. Clarice Laurence, *The Diary of a Flirt* (London, 1915), p. 13.
10. *Daily Mirror*, 27 April 1922, p. 7.
11. Leonard Rossiter, *The Sex Age* (London, 1928), p. 47. See also Herbert Farjeon and Horace Horsnell's play *Advertising April, Or, The Girl Who Made the Sunshine Jealous, A Comedy in* III *Acts* (Oxford, 1922).

12. Robert Graves, *Goodbye to All That* (London, 1928).
13. 'Duped Women', *Manchester Evening News*, 8 October 1915, p. 5; *The Times*, 2 October 1915, p. 3. Fitzgerald was sentenced to eight years in prison.
14. Philip Beaufoy, *Twenty Human Monsters, in Purple and Rags, From Caligula to Landru* (London, 1929), pp. 271 and 273.
15. William Le Queux, *Landru, Bluebeard of France* (London, 1922, repr. 1966), p. 25.
16. Beaufoy, *Twenty Human Monsters*, p. 271.
17. *Daily Mirror*, 3 April 1919, p. 7.
18. *John Bull*, 9 April 1927, p. 22.
19. *Matchmaker*, April 1927, p. 1.
20. *John Bull*, 23 April 1927, p. 14. *Daily Telegraph*, 10 June 1921, p. 3. The UCC operated continuously between 1916 and 1939.
21. *The Times*, 18 May 1928, p. 5. For Moseley's account of the case see Sydney A. Moseley, *The Truth About a Journalist* (London, 1935), pp. 254–55; Moseley, *The Private Diaries of Sydney Moseley* (London, 1960), pp. 290–91. Questions were asked in parliament about the case. See *The Times*, 25 May 1928, p. 8.
22. *The Times*, 18 May 1928, p. 5.
23. For example, the notices from the *Matchmaker* which advertised a 'Gentleman, age 47' wishing to meet 'smart young lady . . . slim, not tall, for companionship only'. Another 'Gentleman' wanted to 'meet good looking lady, under 30 . . . with a view to comradeship on 50-50 basis'. *The Times*, 22 May 1928, p. 5; *Daily Express*, 17 May 1928, p. 11.
24. *Daily Express*, 22 May 1928, p. 11.
25. *Daily Express*, 17 May 1928, p. 11.
26. *The Times*, 17 May 1928, p. 5.
27. *Daily Express*, 18 May 1928, p. 11.
28. *The Times*, 17 May 1928, p. 5.
29. *John Bull*, 30 April 1927, p. 10; *Matchmaker*, July 1928.

30. George Orwell, 'Boys' Weeklies' (1940), in Sonia Orwell and Ian Angus (eds.), *The Collected Essays, Journalism and Letters of George Orwell* (New York, 1968), p. 461.

Chapter 4

1. *The Times*, 31 August 1925.
2. Metropolitan Police Report, 30 September 1925, *Hayley Morriss and Madeleine Roberts, Conspiracy and Offences under the Criminal Law Amendment Act*, TNA MEPO 3/400.
3. Statement of Ethel Stephanie Gray, 31 October 1925, TNA MEPO 3/400.
4. Statement of Sarah Wynne, age 17, of Finsbury Park, 27 October 1925, TNA MEPO 3/400.
5. Statement of Ena Read of Leigh on Sea, 1 November 1925, TNA MEPO 3/400.
6. 'Pippingford Park Trial. 3 Years for Morriss', *Sussex Daily News*, 18 December 1925.
7. 'Crow's Nest Scandal/Hard Labour for Morriss and his Wife', *News of the World*, 20 December 1925, pp. 5–6. A similar case arose in Hove in June 1933 when Eric G-D. advertised for a residential secretary who, amongst other things, had to be a 'good dancer'. He was finally judged to be merely an 'eccentric'. See NVA, *Case Files*, file C173G, Box 118, NVA Collection, Women's Library.
8. On this case, see Judith Walkowitz, *City of Dreadful Delight: Narratives of Sexual Danger in Victorian London* (Chicago, 1992), chs 3 and 4.
9. For NVA correspondence with and delegations to the Home Office, see *Vigilance Record*, March–April 1929, *The Times*, 6 March 1929; *Objectionable Literature Great Britain*, NVA Collection, Women's Library, Box 107 S88H.

10. *MAP, Mainly About People*, 12 February 1910, p. 210; 5 February 1910, p. 177.
11. 'The White Slave Traffic', *MAP*, 12 February 1910, p. 211.
12. Special Report, CID, 7 November 1913, TNA MEPO 3/228, quoted in Paula Bartley, *Prostitution: Prevention and Reform in England 1860–1914* (London, 2000), p. 173.
13. Quoted in Basil Tozer, *The Story of a Terrible Life* (London, 1928), preface.
14. Dr Ninck, Secretary of the Swiss National Vigilance Committee, *Report of the Seventh International Congress for the Suppression of Traffic in Women and Children Held on June 28 to July 1 1927*, 65–67, NVA Collection, Women's Library, Box 108 S88P.
15. Tozer, *Story*, p. 62.
16. Basil Tozer, *Secret Traffic: A Story for the Sophisticated* (London, 1935), p. 9.
17. The figure of 7,000 (not 15,000 as Tozer suggested) women lured into white slavery between 1903 and 1907 came from a misinterpretation of William Coote's assertion that the NVA had met that number of unaccompanied women during that period. See 'The White Slave Traffic', *MAP*, 12 February 1910, p. 211.
18. *Sunday Graphic*, quoted in Tozer, *Story*, front matter.
19. 'Crow's Nest Scandal/Hard Labour for Morriss and his Wife', *News of the World*, 20 December 1925, pp. 5–6.
20. 'The Pippingford Park Case', *Sussex Daily News*, 14 December 1925.
21. Police Report, E. Sussex Constabulary, by John Baker, PC 193, 1 November 1925, TNA MEPO 3/400.
22. Criminal Law Amendment Act 1885, s. 2, cited in indictment against Morriss and Roberts, Calendar for Sussex Assizes, Lewes, 12 December 1925, TNA MEPO 3/400.

Chapter 5

1. Benbow to the Advertising Manager of the *World's Pictorial News*, 30 December 1922, *Benbow and Hyde, Corrupting Public Morals by Selling Obscene Literature*, TNA CRIM 1/234.
2. Estimates of sales can be found in *Appendix to the Home Office Confidential Circular letter of 8th April 1938 sent to Chief Constables*, TNA CUST 49/233; C. P. Hill, *Report to the Home Office*, January 1939, TNA HO 45/24761.
3. Proceedings Against Obscene Publications in England and Wales, *Report of the Inter-Departmental Working Party on Obscene Publications* 1951, TNA HO 302/12.
4. Mervyn Hyde to Cyril Benbow, 7 January 1923, *Benbow and Hyde, Corrupting Public Morals by Selling Obscene Literature*, TNA CRIM 1/234.
5. Hyde to Benbow, undated, TNA CRIM 1/234.
6. Ibid.
7. Hyde's diary, TNA CRIM 1/234.
8. Statement of William Benbow, 18 April 1923, TNA CRIM 1/234. On the market at this time see Lisa Sigel, *Governing Pleasures: Pornography and Social Change in Britain 1815–1914* (New York, 2003).
9. *R v Hicklin* (1868), quoted in Colin Manchester, 'A History of the Crime of Obscene Libel', *Journal of Legal History*, 12, 1 (May 1991), pp. 36–57, p. 47.
10. See police evidence to *Joint Select Committee on Lotteries and Indecent Advertisements 1908*, Parliamentary Papers (1908), 275, ix 375.
11. Harold Brainerd Hersey, *Pulpwood Editor: The Fabulous World of the Thriller Magazines Revealed by a Veteran Editor and Publisher* (New York, 1937), p. vii. Sales figures estimated by the Home Office based on comparison with the sales of *Razzle*, then a humour pulp, quoted by Alexander MacLaren, Secretary of the National Federation of Retail Newsagents, Booksellers and Stationers, to J. F. Henderson, 2 May 1934, TNA MEPO 3/2323. One art

studies title was said to sell 143,000 worldwide. See 'French Magazines Condemned', *The Times*, 3 February 1937, p. 11. For a more detailed discussion, see H. G. Cocks, 'Saucy Stories: Pornography, Sexology and the Marketing of Sexual Knowledge in Britain, c. 1918–1970', *Social History*, 29, 4 (November 2004): pp. 465–87.

12. See CID Report, 14 April 1937, *Indecent Literature By Post: Leonard William Steer*, TNA MEPO 3/938; 'Photographs Alleged to be Indecent, Prosecution of Small Heath Man', *Birmingham Post*, 28 October 1927.
13. Evidence of Chief Inspector Edward Drew, *Joint Select Committee on Lotteries and Indecent Advertisements 1908*, PP. (1908), 275, ix 375, pp. 431–32.
14. Evidence of W. P. Burn, Asst. Under Secretary of State at Home Dept, *Joint Select Committee on Lotteries and Indecent Advertisements 1908*, p. 414.
15 C. H. Rafter, Chief Constable of Warwickshire, to Secretary of State, 10 January 1908, *Sale of Abortifacients by Post*, TNA HO 10932/15.
16. *Fun*, 4 and 11 June 1921.
17. 'Do Wantons Dress Immodestly?', *London Life and Modern Society*, 10 January 1920, p. 11.
18. *London Life*, 21 December 1929, p. 67.
19. Benbow to R. E. Matheson, 13 March 1923, TNA CRIM 1/234.
20. 'An Appreciation', *London Life*, 1 January 1921, p. 13.
21. Alec Craig, *The Banned Books of England* (London, 1937), pp. 154 and 155.

Chapter 6

1. On the rubber-goods/obscene book industry and the Economy Educator see Roy Porter and Lesley Hall, *The Facts of Life: The Creation of Sexual Knowledge in Britain, 1650–1950* (New Haven,

1995), ch. 11. Hall concludes that 'A continued association between informative sex manual and pornography throughout this period can be deduced'. *Facts of Life*, p. 263. On Economy Educator see Lesley Hall, *Sex, Gender and Social Change in Britain Since 1880* (London, 2000), p. 137.

2. Gradations of obscenity, especially in postcards, did inform police procedure. In general, nudes in themselves were not indecent, 'but partially dressed females . . . in suggestive poses were definitely indecent.' Police Report, March 1933, *Cases of Indecent Literature, 1932–34*, PRO HO 45/24939. See also Frederick Hallis, *The Law and Obscenity* (London, 1932), p. 17.
3. 'An Encyclopaedia of Sexual Knowledge', *British Medical Journal*, 14 July 1934, pp. 94–95, p. 95.
4. Letter from Norman Haire, *British Medical Journal*, 12 July 1934, p. 152.
5. Walter M. Gallichan, *The Poison of Prudery: An Historical Survey* (London, 1929), p. 147.
6. Alec Craig, *Above All Liberties* (London, 1942), p. 103.
7. *London Life*, 8 January 1921, p. 15; 15 January 1921, p. 15.
8. *Business Chances* 2, 6 (October–November 1934), p. 4.
9. Advertisement for Panurge Press, *Ballyhoo*, January 1934, p. 30 Panurge sold Jacobus X's compendious 1890s account of colonial sexology, *Untrodden Fields of Anthropology*, alongside the works of Bloch, Hirschfeld and other sexologists. Panurge sent books to the British empire as well. See Home Office file and Panurge Press Circular (undated), 1935, TNA HO 45/20913. The British pulp *Razzle* also advertised books like Winfield Scott Hall's *Sexual Knowledge* (London, 1933), see *Razzle*, February 1933.
10. Opinion of Sir Edward Tindal Atkinson, quoted in *Minutes of Evidence Taken Before the Select Committee on the Obscene Publications Bill*, Parl. Papers, 1957–58 (122) vol. vi. pp. 441 and 664. The opinion was given in 1936.

11. Statement of Geoffrey Edwin Keith Worsfield of 17 Sunnywood Drive, Haywards Heath, Sussex, Shop Assistant, age 29, 15 December 1950, *Park Trading*, TNA MEPO 2/9132.
12. Statement of Walter Voysey Scanes, 52, of Wallington, Surrey, 14 December 1950, MEPO 2/9132.
13. 'Photographs Alleged to be Indecent, Prosecution of Small Heath Man', *Birmingham Post*, 28 October 1927.
14. Direct Book Supply Catalogue, undated, 1949. Mass Observation, University of Sussex, TC 12 Box 16 File A. See also Porter and Hall, *Facts of Life*, pp. 262–63.
15. Kate Fisher, *Birth Control, Sex and Marriage in Britain, 1918–1960* (Oxford, 2006).
16. Police Report, E. Sussex Constabulary, by DC Vernon Paris, 15 December 1950, *Park Trading*, TNA MEPO 2/9132.
17. Statement of John Harrin Evans, of 24 Bridgend St, Cardiff, a steel worker at Dowlais works, 21 December 1950, TNA MEPO 2/9132.

CHAPTER 7

1. Mary Oliver and Mary Benedetta, *Marriage Bureau* (London, 1942), p. 19.
2. Ibid.
3. Heather Jenner, *Marriage is My Business* (London, 1953), p. 13.
4. National Marriage Guidance Council, *Report to the Executive Committee of the NMGC From its Committee of Inquiry into Marriage Agencies*, March 1949, TNA HO 45/25203.
5. Oliver and Benedetta, *Marriage Bureau*, p. 28.
6. 'Pay £5 5s and Wait for Husband', *Daily Mail*, 14 April 1939, p. 11; 'Debs Tired of the "Bright Young Men" They Meet', *Daily Mail*, 18 April 1939, p. 11; 'Godfrey Winn's Page', *Sunday Express*, 23 April 1939, p. 19.

7. Helen Berry, *Gender, Society and Print Culture in Late-Stuart England: The Cultural World of the Athenian Mercury* (Aldershot, 2003).
8. Anon., *Matrimonial Advertisements*, Private Collection, 1740–1859, British Library.
9. Ibid.
10. J. Curtis, *An Authentic and Faithful History of the Mysterious Murder of Maria Marten* (London, 1828).
11. William Booth, *In Darkest England and the Way Out* (London, 1890), pp. 233–36.
12. V. F. Calverton, *The Bankruptcy of Marriage* (London, 1929).
13. Mean age of marriage of all single men and women, Office of National Statistics, National Statistics Online, www.statistics.gov.uk (12 May 2008).
14. On these, see Catherine Gasquoine Hartley, 'The Sexes Again', *English Review*, September 1913, pp. 268–83; *Motherhood and the Relationship of the Sexes* (London, 1917).
15. On these, see Gasquoine Hartley, 'The Sexes Again'.
16. Gasquoine Hartley, 'The Sexes Again', p. 226, and Catherine Gasquoine Hartley, 'Marriage a Racial Duty', *Lloyd's Weekly News*, 22 March 1920, p. 8.
17. Clement Wood, *Why I Believe in Trial Marriage* (Girard, Kan. 1929); Leonard Rossiter, *The Sex Age* (London, 1928).
18. Ben B. Lindsay, *The Companionate Marriage* (London, 1928).
19. J. A. Goldsmid, *Companionate Marriage From the Medical and Social Aspects* (London, 1934), p. 13.
20. The best history of the NMGC is Jane Lewis, David Clark and David H. J. Morgan, '*Whom God Hath Joined Together': The Work of Marriage Guidance* (London, 1992).
21. A. H. Halsey and Josephine Webb (eds), *Twentieth Century British Social Trends* (Basingstoke, 2000), p. 62; B. R. Mitchell, *British Historical Statistics* (Cambridge, 1988), p. 76.
22. Wenzell Brown, *Introduction to Murder* (New York, 1951).

23. 'Star Fan Club', *Picture Show*, 22 January 1949; Obituary of Alec Bregonzi, *Guardian*, 9 June 2006.
24. Barry Johnston, *Johnners: The Life of Brian* (London, 2003), pp. 153–54.
25. *Friendship Clubs, Mass Observation*, University of Sussex, TC 12 Box 16 File E.
26. Alan Wykes, *The Pen-Friend* (London, 1950); Angus Wilson, *Hemlock and After* (London, 1952). Many thanks to Vincent Quinn for the latter reference.
27. 'The Marriage Business', *Sunday Pictorial*, 28 March 1948, p. 5.
28. Ibid.
29. David Mace, *Marriage Crisis* (London, 1948), p. 7.
30. David Mace, 'A Specialist's report on agencies that help people in the Search For a Life Partner', *John Bull*, 20 March 1948, p. 6; Minutes of the AGM of NMGC, 19 May 1949, Marriage Agencies, *National Marriage Guidance Council: Report on Matrimonial Agencies*, 1948–9, TNA HO 45/25203.
31. Ibid. p. 6; Harvey Graham, 'Preparing for Marriage', *John Bull*, 15 May 1948; Minutes of the AGM of NMGC, 19 May 1949, Marriage Agencies, *National Marriage Guidance Council: Report on Matrimonial Agencies*, 1948–9, TNA HO 45/25203.
32. 'Free Speech: Matrimony', *John Bull*, 20 March 1948, p. 15.
33. 'The Answer to the Marriage Muddle', *Sunday Pictorial*, 18 April 1948, p. 4.
34. Note of W. M. Goode, 27 July 1949, *National Marriage Guidance Council: Report on Matrimonial Agencies, 1948–9*, TNA HO 45/25203.
35. Note of P. Boysmith, 12 June 1949, *National Marriage Guidance Council: Report on Matrimonial Agencies, 1948–9*, TNA HO 45/25203.
36. *Report to the Executive Committee of the NMGC From its Committee of Inquiry into Marriage Agencies*, March 1949, p. 14; *National Marriage Guidance Council: Report on Matrimonial Agencies, 1948–9*, TNA HO 45/25203.

37. John Gillis sees the 1950s as the culmination of an age of 'compulsory marriage' dating back to 1850. See Gillis, *For Better, For Worse*, chs 8 and 9.
38. Mean age at marriage of all single men marrying single women, National Statistics Online, www.statistics.gov.uk (12 May 2008).

CHAPTER 8

1. *Exit*, 38 (1968).
2. Ibid.
3. Statement of Reginald Brothers, Det. Sgt. New Scotland Yard, 18 November 1968. Central Criminal Court Autumn sessions, 1969, DPP, Copy of Statements Tendered in Evidence, *Donelly and Mcguigan,* Exit *and* Way Out, *Conspiracy to corrupt Public Morals*, TNA DPP 2/4598.
4. 'Ladies' Directory: Summonses', *The Times*, 27 July 1960, p. 8; 'Ladies' Directory: Convictions and Sentence Stand', *The Times*, 15 December 1960, p. 13. Thanks to David Cocks for a discussion of this case and many references.
5. Richard Gardner, 'How Good are Your Orgasms? Magical Love Making', *IT*, 20, October 27–November 9 1967, p. 3.
6. Emmanuel Petrakis, 'The Sexual Revolution', *IT* 14–27 February 1969, pp. 12–13.
7. Yippie pamphlet, quoted in Richard Neville, *Play Power* (London, 1970), p. 57.
8. Fred Vermorel, *Fashion and Perversity: A Life of Vivienne Westwood and the Sixties Laid Bare* (London, 1996), p. 150.
9. *IT*, 20, October 27–November 9 1967, p. 16.
10. *Jeffrey*, 2 (1973), p. 21.
11. *Exit*, no. 38 (undated, prob. 1968), *Donelly and McGuigan, Donelly and Mcguigan,* 'Exit' *and* 'Way Out'*: Conspiracy to corrupt Public Morals*, TNA DPP 2/4598.

12. Jonathon Green, *All Dressed Up: The Sixties and the Counterculture* (London, 1999), p. 332.
13. Edward M. Brecher, *The Sex Researchers* (London, 1970), p. 273; Thomas J. B. and Everett Myers, *Wife Swapping* (New York, 1965), pp. 149–50.
14. Michael Leigh, *The Velvet Underground* (1963); Matt Galant, *Mate-Swapping Syndrome* (1967); Christopher Storm, *The Sex Rebels* (1964).
15. 'Group Sex: Is it "Life Art" or a Sign That Something is Wrong?', *New York Times*, 10 May 1971, p. 38.
16. Brecher, *Sex Researchers*, pp. 247–48. The major ones were *Ecstasy*, *Latent Image*, *Kindred Spirits*, *Swingers' Life*, *La Plume*, *Kit Kat*, *Select*, *Rebel*, *Swing*, *National Informer*, *20th Century Club*, *Club Infinite*, *Kismet Society*, *Club Joy*, *Communique*, *Renaissance Club*, *'Sharon'*, *American Club*, *Club Accolade*, *The Swinging World*, *National Registry*, *Hot Line*, *Clique*, and assorted girlie magazines and underground papers like the *LA Free Press* and *IT*. See William and Jerrye Breedlove, *Swap Clubs: A Study in Contemporary Sexual Mores* (Los Angeles, 1964); Richard Warren Lewis, 'The Swingers', *Playboy*, 16, 4 (April 1969), pp. 149–50, 216–28, p. 150. See note 26 for British titles.
17. Swingers' ads, source not given, quoted in Gilbert D. Bartell, *Group Sex: A Scientist's Report on the American Way of Swinging* (New York, 1971), p. 85.
18. Brecher, *Sex Researchers*, p. 249.
19. Richard Warren Lewis, 'The Swingers', *Playboy*, 16, 4 (April 1969), pp. 149–50, 216–28.
20. Bartell, *Group Sex*, pp. 34–42.
21. Lewis, 'The Swingers', p. 150.
22. Bartell, *Group Sex*, pp. 19–20.
23. Ibid. p. 43.
24. Ibid. p. 50.
25. Ibid. pp. 81–82.

26. That is, if you include gay magazines. In addition to *Jeffrey*, the other main gay magazine was the *Jeffrey* spin-off, *Rugged Male*. The swingers' mags, some of which had a very home-made look about them were *Exit*, *Way Out*, *International Way Out*, *Contact*, *International Personal Advertiser*, *Adult Advertiser*, *Adds And*, *New Friends* and *Blue Circle*, *The Correspondent* and *La Plume*, some of which may have been the same paper under different titles. *The Correspondent* claimed 20,000 readers. *Correspondent*, 18 (1969), editorial, p. 1. Some *Exit* users also used the other magazines, see Statement of Reginald Brothers, DS 19 Feb 1969, TNA DPP 2/4598.
27. Christine Keeler with Douglas Thompson, *The Truth at Last: My Story* (London, 2002), pp. 43–45.
28. Clive Irving, Ron Hall, Jeremy Wallington, *Scandal '63* (London, 1963), p. 226.
29. Indictment, Transcript of Appeal, House of Lords, 11 June 1972, TNA DPP 2/4598.
30. CID report by DS Brothers, 19 February 1969, TNA DPP 2/4598.
31. Elkan Allan, *Love in Our Time, With an Introduction by Eustace Chesser; compiled and edited by Donald Wiedenman from the original research interviews with Elkan Allan* (London, 1968).
32. 'Why I Made "Love In Our Time",' *Sunday People*, 10 November 1968, pp. 2–3.
33. Letter of Michael L., (undated), TNA DPP 2/4598.
34. Letter of Michael L.; Letter of Richard, 12 November 1968, TNA DPP 2/4598.
35. Eustace Chesser, introduction to Elkan Allan, *Love In Our Time* (London, 1968); Brecher, Sex Researchers, p. 270.
36. 'Your Verdict on That Film', *Sunday People*, 17 November 1968, p. 14.
37. Neville, *Play Power*, p. 58.
38. Green, *All Dressed Up*, p. 331.

39. Quoted in Brecher, *Sex Researchers*, p. 228.
40. *Time Out*, September 1971, p. 58.

Epilogue

1. Manuel Castells, *The Rise of the Network Society* (Oxford, 1996).
2. Castells, *Network Society*, p. 328.
3. Sherry Turkle, *Life on the Screen: Identity in the Age of the Internet* (New York, 1995).
4. Sadie Plant, 'Coming Across the Future', in David Bell and Barbara M. Kennedy, *The Cybercultures Reader* (London, 2000), pp. 460–61.
5. Aaron Ben Ze'ev, *Love Online: Emotions on the Internet* (Cambridge, 2004), pp. 26 and 27.
6. Jeffrey Boase and Barry Wellman, 'Personal Relationships: On and Off the Internet', in Anita L. Vangelisti and Daniel Perlman, (eds), *The Cambridge Handbook of Personal Relationships* (Cambridge, 2006), pp. 709–23.
7. *A Guide to Modern Romance, Observer/ITV1* pull-out section March 2007, pp. 20–21.
8. 'Flirting and Fornicating', *Guardian*, 23 July 2007; 'Love by Numbers', *Guardian Weekend*, 10 November 2007, p. 117.
9. *Guardian*, 23 July 2007.
10. 'Let's Talk About Sex', *Guardian*, 17 February 2007; 'Sex, now', *Guardian*, 15 April 2006.
11. According to Esther Addley's 2007 article, 'Gay bars and gay areas in major cities have felt its impact – an article in the Economist last year attributed a downturn in the fortunes of Manchester's famous Canal Street gay quarter directly to Gaydar'. 'Let's Talk About Sex', *Guardian*, 17 February 2007; 'Cruising in Style', *Guardian*, 31 July 2006.

12. 'Sensuality a Must in Tangled Web of Love', *Guardian*, 8 December 2004.
13. 'Seeking Romance: GSOH and Web 2.0 Compatibility Essential', *Guardian*, 12 July 2007.
14. 'Looking for Love, but Used for Sex', *Guardian*, 6 November 2006.
15. University of Bath, Press Release, 14 February 2005, www.bath.ac.uk/pr/releases/internet-dating.htm (15 June 2008).
16. Andrew Keen, quoted in *Observer*, 29 April 2007, p. 3, see also Keen, *The Cult of the Amateur, or How Today's Internet is Killing our Culture and Assaulting Our Economy* (London, 2007).
17. Stephanie Coontz, *Marriage, A History: How Love Conquered Marriage* (London, 2006).
18. 'The End of Marriage', *Observer Magazine*, 2 March 2008, p. 36.
19. Umberto Eco, *The Name of the Rose* (New York, 1982), preface.
20. *Guardian*, 1 September 2006, p. 1.
21. 'Seeking Romance', *Guardian*, 12 July 2007.
22. 'Romance Makes a Comeback in the Dating Game', *Guardian*, 12 February 2005.
23. David Weinberger, quoted in Nicholas Lemann, 'Amateur Hour', *The New Yorker*, 7 August 2006.
24. *Link*, July 1916, p. 2.

Details about Advertisements Displayed in the Text

Introduction

p. ix Anon, *Matrimonial Advertisements* (*c.* 1740–1859) 1750

Chapter 1

p. 4 *Link*, June 1919
p. 6 *Link*, June 1919
p. 9 *T. P.'s Weekly*, 26 April 1912, p. 540
p. 17 *Round-About*, 2 July 1898, p. 11
p. 20 *T. P.'s Weekly*, 2 January 1914, p. 60
p. 21 *T. P.'s Weekly*, 2 January 1914, p. 91

Chapter 2

p. 29 *T. P.'s Weekly*, 12 February 1916, p. 166
p. 31 *T. P.'s Weekly*, 12 February 1916, p. 166
p. 35 *T. P.'s Weekly*, 12 February 1916, p. 166
p. 38 *T. P.'s Weekly*, 12 February 1916, p. 166

Chapter 3

p. 46 *Morning Post*, 22 December 1921
p. 50 *The Times*, 2 October 1915, p. 3

p. 51 *Matchmaker*, January 1928, p. 3
p. 57 *Matchmaker*, quoted in *The Times*, 22 May 1928

Chapter 4

p. 64 *The Times*, 31 August 1925
p. 70 *T. P.'s Weekly*, 22 September 1911, p. 380
p. 74 *MAP, Mainly about People*, 12 February 1910, p. 210
p. 77 Quoted in *John Bull*, 30 April 1927, p. 10
p. 79 *T. P.'s Weekly*, 5 May 1911, p. 574

Chapter 5

p. 88 *Business Chances*, September–October 1936, p. 1
p. 93 *Business Chances*, December–January 1935–36, inside back cover
p. 98 *London Life*, 15 January 1921

Chapter 6

p. 105 *London Life*, 6 July 1929
p. 109 *Business Chances*, June–July 1935, p. 22
p. 113 Circular distributed in Reading, 1931, British Library TNA HO 45/15753
p. 116 *My Pocket Novels*, 1074, 1922

Chapter 7

p. 121 *Matchmaker*, January 1928, p. 2
p. 123 *Matchmaker*, January 1928, p. 6
p. 127 *The Times*, 22 May 1928
p. 131 *Writer*, May 1949

p. 133 Quoted in *Sunday Pictorial*, 28 March 1948, p. 5

p. 138 Quoted in *Sunday Pictorial*, 28 March 1948, p. 5

Chapter 8

p. 145 *Exit*, 38, 1968

p. 151 *Correspondent* 19, 1969

p. 157 Quoted in Bartell, *Group Sex* (*c.* 1969–70), p. 85

p. 162 *Correspondent* 19, 1969

p. 169 *Correspondent* 19, 1969

p. 172 *Correspondent* 19, 1969

Index